YOUR MIND BUILDS YOUR BODY

Unlock Your Potential with Biohacking
and Strength Training

Your Mind Builds Your Body
Roger Snipes

First published in the UK and USA in 2021 by
Watkins, an imprint of Watkins Media Limited
Unit 11, Shepperton House
89–93 Shepperton Road
London N1 3DF

enquiries@watkinspublishing.com

COMMISSIONING EDITOR: Etan Ilfeld
MANAGING EDITOR: Daniel Culver
DEVELOPMENT EDITOR: Anya Hayes
HEAD OF DESIGN: Glen Wilkins
PRODUCTION: Uzma Taj
ASSOCIATE NUTRITIONIST: Riya Lakhani (ANutr)

A CIP record for this book is available from the British Library.

ISBN: 978-1-78678-448-3 (paperback)

ISBN: 978-1-78678-476-6 (eBook)

10 9 8 7 6 5 4 3 2 1

Set in Trajan and Gotham

Printed in Turkey

www.watkinspublishing.com

Publisher's note: The information in this book is not intended as a substitute for professional medical advice and treatment. If you are pregnant or are suffering from any medical conditions or health problems, it is recommended that you consult a medical professional before following any of the advice or practice suggested in this book. Watkins Media Limited, or any other persons who have been involved in working on this publication, cannot accept responsibility for any injuries or damage incurred as a result of following the information, exercises or therapeutic techniques contained in this book.

YOUR MIND BUILDS YOUR BODY

Unlock Your Potential with Biohacking and Strength Training

Roger Snipes

with Daniel Culver

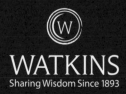

WATKINS
Sharing Wisdom Since 1893

CONTENTS

*CP# (Core Principles)

HOW TO USE THIS BOOK

Think of this book as a toolbox presented in four easy-to-navigate parts.

Part 1 follows my own unique journey into the fitness industry. How an interest in sprinting led me to bodybuilding, which fuelled a personal desire to improve my own physique, and how that then led me to where I am today.

Part 2 explores the impact of mind over matter. How looking after our own mental health can benefit our bodies. Building self-confidence is as important as building muscle. Trust me, these two go hand in hand.

Part 3 look at the body. I explore biology and the impact of science on bodybuilding. I also explore genetics and nutrition, and how to get the most from your own bodies, including many of the biohacking techniques that I use within my own programme.

Part 4 will help you structure a training programme unique to your own needs. I present the exercise routines I swear by. Simple lifts and hacks, along with hints and tips that you can use in and out of the gym. This includes creating a meal plan, and the different types of diets ...

🎙 Along the way you will find the podcast icon beside sections that are explored on my podcast, *The Roger Snipes Show*, should you wish to dive deeper into a subject area:

beacons.ai/therogersnipesshow

*Disclaimer: If in doubt, consult your doctor.
Know your limits. Becoming injured will only further impede your training. Dieting too hard will likewise have adverse effects on your wellbeing. Start slow and continue steady. This is not a race. It's a chance to reset.

INTRODUCTION

This is an extensive exercise and lifestyle guide for men who want something a little bit special – a plan that sits outside of the usual cookie-cutter, one-size-fits-all, get-fit-quick programmes that are perpetuated within the fitness industry.

Instead, this guide outlines a detailed syllabus for improving mind and body and is suitable for all levels, ages and abilities.

We will explore at what's inside – the things that make us tick – before we progress to the fundamentals of the body and the science behind exercise and bodybuilding.

The programme includes:

›› **Insight into the psychology of bodybuilding.**

›› **Brain health: how training your mind is just as important as training your muscles.**

›› **In-depth advice and guidance on nutrition and supplements.**

›› **A break down on various dietary techniques, including the science behind fat loss and muscle gain.**

›› **Comprehensive meal plans to maximize your training.**

›› **Advanced biohacking techniques and the scientific research behind them.**

›› **Alternative, non-tech biohacking strategies to optimize your health and strength.**

›› **Techniques to transform your physical and mental confidence and practice, including mindfulness, breathing and programme planning.**

›› **Tips and plans to keep you on track and how to avoid derailing your entire programme for the sake of one slip up, particularly around holidays or at Christmas (when life gets in the way).**

›› **Alternative biohacking techniques.**

›› **Simple but effective exercises and bodybuilding routines that you can follow at home, or in the gym, meaning you don't need to spend large amounts of money to improve yourself.**

This book is a complete blueprint to improve mindset and physical potential.

It is not just a quick-fit remedy for transformation and I do not claim to be able to give you a beach body in 8–12 weeks, though if you follow the protocols that I have laid out for you, you will acquire the necessary tools to greatly improve your health and wellbeing and with it your physique.

A good diet and training regime might get you a six-pack, but you will need to instill good habits to keep yourself lean and in shape. And habits are of course formed in the mind.

You don't need luck, or good genes, you just need discipline. You need to retrain your mind.

All of the things I present in this book can be learned and applied by anyone, anywhere and all you need is some basic kit and a set of self-imposed rules to keep you on track.

Mindset Tools and Fitness Rules

When we think about health and fitness, we tend to think about exercise and food. We think about rules and regimes. What we tend to ignore though are other factors that can profoundly affect the body's ability to perform. The science behind what we are doing. Hidden obstacles such as stress, mental health and low testosterone – and any number of internal obstacles that can inhibit muscle growth, energy and strength. Particularly in men of a certain age.

Stress is in essence a sickness within the mind. It is perhaps the most detrimental thing to our health and wellbeing, but men especially seem to either overlook their mental wellbeing or disregard it altogether. How then does stress cause an imbalance within the body? How do hormones work? How does blood sugar affect our biology in terms of health and fitness? What impact does DNA have on genetic potential? And how can light and electromagnetic fields affect the way we sleep, feel and perform both in and out of the gym?

Fitness is about knowledge and adaptation.
The more insight you gain, the more tools you
have, the more problems you can solve.
The better you can become.

While this book does explore the fundamentals of weight training and nutrition, it is not your typical book about bodybuilding and diet.

I'm here to offer a fresh perspective on fitness and present a guide that goes a little further than "eat this, lift that, and then repeat the cycle for twelve weeks".

I plan to give you tools you can use to re-programme your mindset and your body for the long haul.

Why are you here?

Maybe you're here because you're interested in my story. Or perhaps you want to find out about my meal prep, training schedule, or my body part split. Maybe you're here because your own training has stalled, and you're looking for clarification, or just plain old inspiration.

I can't promise miracles, but I will aim to present you with the things I have learned over the 20+ years I have been training. In that time, I've worked with experts in the field of nutrition and science; this includes supplement companies, dieticians, athletes, bodybuilders and fitness professionals from all over the world, as well as the many clients that I've personally trained.

Where do we begin?

In the pages that follow, I aim to pool all of the things that I have learned over the course of many years – building a physique that has opened many doors for me – and present you with what I feel are the fundamental building blocks of fitness. This should equip you with the appropriate knowledge, enabling you to determine what is right and wrong for you. Giving you the tools to tailor your own programme; something that fits around your life and commitments.

My intention is not to give you a template to follow. You can find a hundred of these online, and for free, and if you follow them to a T you will probably see some improvements. Instead, I want to present you with a dynamic blueprint for total mind and body transformation. Practical advice that will stay with you for life.

But this isn't a one-size-fits-all instruction manual. Everybody and every body type is different, and so too is every mind. There is no blanket fix that will work the same for everyone. Likewise, there are not enough pages in this book to list every individual option, opinion, route, plan or programme, though I will try to give you the fundamentals of my own plan – things I swear by, and some things I swear against – and you can take or leave them as you wish.

We all have different reasons for wanting to overhaul our lives. It may be health related, or it might be vanity. There's nothing wrong with wanting to look and feel good. You shouldn't wait around for something bad to happen before you make that change in your life.

But please bear in mind: **everyone's starting blocks begin in different spots**, so what may work just fine for one person may be detrimental to another. Don't compare yourself to other people. I've been blessed in that I've never had any traumatic sicknesses or any lasting injuries. I'm not bulletproof – by any means – but I still work at it; I still do whatever I can to keep strong and healthy. And now I want to pass my ethos along to you.

Together we will look at genetics and the fundamentals of the body, including testosterone levels and how this can affect men of a certain age. And, more vitally, how low T-levels can be improved, not just through diet or by lifting heavy weights, but via alternative methods.

I then want us look at diets and explore why some work while others may not, factoring in age, body type, ability and, of course, time.

We will also explore biohacking, and will present you with easy to understand, advanced scientific methods that you can add as an accompaniment to your daily plan, in order to enhance you both physically and mentally. This book will help you become the best version of you – in both body and in brain!

In addition to my tried and tested training methods, I will also explore all aspects of training – whether that is for the casual gym goer, budding bodybuilders, professional athletes, or for the complete beginner and leave you with a plan you can tailor to meet your needs.

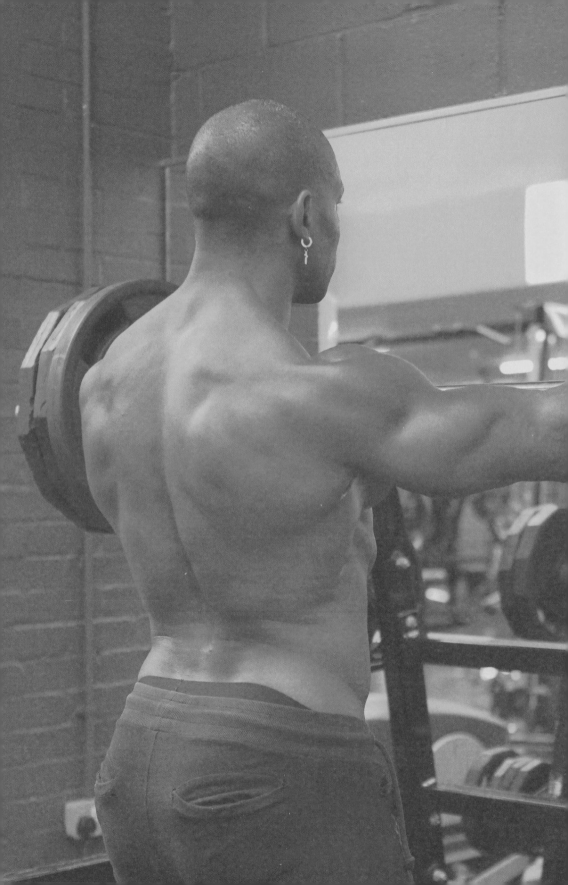

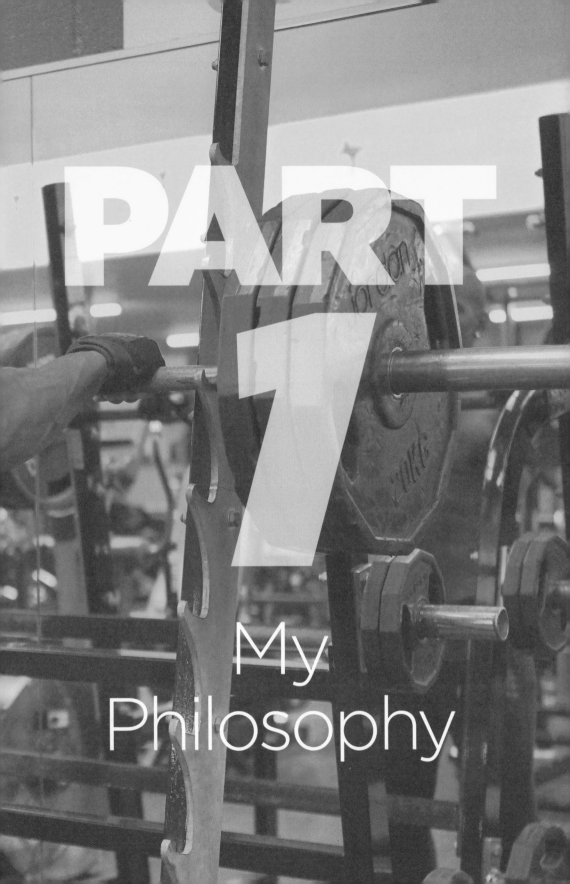

PART

1

My
Philosophy

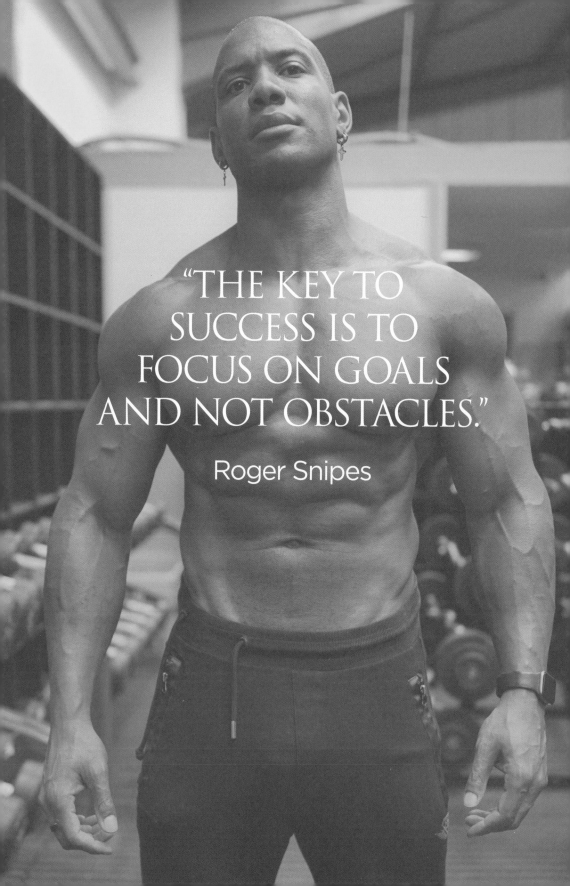

"THE KEY TO SUCCESS IS TO FOCUS ON GOALS AND NOT OBSTACLES."

Roger Snipes

CHAPTER 1

THE REAL ROGER SNIPES

Let me start by giving you a brief insight into who I am and what got me here. What I'm all about. Why I chose to dedicate my life to the pursuit of the perfect physique, and what drove the choices and decisions that I made along the way.

Here, I will discuss my philosophies and lifestyle choices. Why I opted to remain natural, and I'm not just talking synthetics, but also organic produce, steering clear of manmade products and protein powders, for the most part. To begin with, I will look at the most overlooked and undertrained muscle: the brain. How do our minds factor into our training regimes? In what way does mindfulness benefit the body under training conditions and how does it enable us to better control our health, optimizing wellbeing, as well?

I will of course look at nutrition, also. This includes the overall benefits of clean, healthy eating and why I chose to reject the typical bodybuilding route, opting instead for one of scientific discovery. I will discuss the dietary choices I have make and the things I have changed along the way due to improved knowledge and experience. I will also show you how important biohacking is and how it has become a part of my daily routine (*see* Chapter 8).

Finally, we will take an in-depth look at the unique training programme I have created in search of optimal health and peak fitness. I will share the exercises and hacks that have helped me transition from athletics to bodybuilding to fitness entrepreneur, and the things I do to maintain my own physique.

This will equip you with everything I believe you need to achieve your own ultimate body.

I'm in my 40s, which means that more than half of my life has been spent in pursuit of peak health. I've been fine-tuning my physique since I was a teenager, and while I've made great gains, I've also made mistakes along the way. I believe these things – both good and bad – are vital in order to learn what works and what does not. I have also consulted experts in science and nutrition, and fellow specialists in the field of biohacking to bring you the ultimate How To Guide.

My Story

My fascination with fitness and the human form began at a very young age. I was born competitive. Some of my earliest memories are of running through the streets of North London, where I grew up. My competitive streak began there, with simple street games like tag or knock down ginger. Like most young boys, living on an estate where there was not much else to do, my friends and I would actively look for trouble to pass the time. Getting chased by the police became a pastime of sorts, especially for my friends, though for me it was another challenge; even back then when we were setting of fireworks or kicking in doors and running away, I was looking to test my speed. It was the same with every sport I played. Football, for example, was never my forte – I wasn't very skilful with the ball – but I always strived to be the fastest on the field. Being the *fastest* was what interested me and so I was always in competition, with my friends and with myself.

That's when I discovered I had a real talent for running. I have no idea why, but I was obsessed with being as fast and as fit as possible. I knew even back then that those who work at perfecting their craft have more chance of becoming experts or professionals, and I could feel myself being drawn in that direction.

The Power of Positive Influences

It's important to seek out inspiration when you are beginning your fitness journey. I'm lucky to have had real mentors later on, but starting out I was alone and so I looked for positive role models. There were few men I idolised as much as Linford Christie and Arnold Schwarzenegger. When Linford came to the forefront of British Athletics in the 1980s and 90s, he became one of my first idols and was the first athlete I really identified with. Here was this great black, British sprinter who was not only lightning quick, but was also in incredible shape. His physique was perfect. So muscular, and he carried himself with such confidence. As soon as I heard him being interviewed on television about his regimen – a programme that involved more than just sprint training, but also included weight training and a special diet – that's when it all clicked. That's when I thought: *I need to get myself in shape like him.*

And so, it began. As my sprint time improved, I started to focus on my appearance as well. I wanted to stand out. I wanted a body that would show my hard-earned efforts. It was around this time that I discovered Arnold Schwarzenegger. I remember being completely blown away by his physique and thought, oh my god, who is this guy? I couldn't even pronounce his name, but I was mesmerized by the way he looked. He had an amazing presence and determination, which I admired, and like Linford Christie he became a great inspiration to me.

These men inspired me, so when people tell me that I've inspired them in much the same way, that really is an amazing feeling.

And so, inspired by my new idols I began to do simple workouts in my bedroom. At first, this involved basic push-ups and bodyweight squats. I would also run around the park, putting myself through sprinting drills, doing shuttle runs, and other practices to increase my speed. Things I still swear by today.

THE REAL ROGER SNIPES

FINDING MY WAY

There was a lot of crime in my neighbourhood. My dad didn't trust anyone on the estate where we lived, and he didn't want me to be outside with my friends because he knew we were getting up to no good. So, as a compromise, he got me my first set of weights. I was about nine years old and like most people toying with bodybuilding, I didn't know what the hell I was doing. I was blindly trying to find my way. My dad was not into training himself, but I think he was glad that my new-found interest in fitness had taken my focus away from crime, even though I had no clue what I was doing.

THE TURNING POINT

I saw what was going on in my neighbourhood. I had friends who were either getting stabbed or arrested, so I spent a lot of my teenage years indoors. It was there that I became dedicated to the idea of becoming super-fit, as well as super-fast. I wanted to build a formidable body. It took time, but soon friends began to notice the transformation. People began telling me I was looking "kind-of big". That gave me a boost, and it wasn't long before I noticed the difference myself.

I wasn't making money like my friends were: some were out on the streets robbing and hustling, others had well-off parents, so they got decent pocket money. Meanwhile, I was still getting £1 a week from my Dad and I had to make that last. I'd save up to buy myself a fitness magazine once a month. That was like my bible. Reading those magazines from cover to cover, I would absorb all of the information, follow the workouts inside, and then try to incorporate all of the different exercises into my own programme in the hope I could get even bigger and stronger and take my fitness to the next level.

By the age of 16, I was obsessed. I was attending every fitness class that I could, including Spin and Body Pump. I was young and naive, and hungry to learn. But that's how it began.

"ACCEPT EVERY LOSS AS AN OPPORTUNITY TO LEARN. THAT WAY YOU ALWAYS WIN."

Roger Snipes

POWER THROUGH IMPOSTER SYNDROME 🎙

I know so many people feel anxious when they first begin working out. It's that fear of picking up a weight, or entering the gym for the first time and looking clueless. I've been there too. That sense of imposter syndrome: being new and knowing nothing. You're not alone. I guarantee, everyone in the gym has felt this at some point. Myself included. But the only way through is through.

COMPETITION

In my 20s, I looked at fitness magazines similar to those I had bought with my pocket money as a teenager, with a new perspective and more years of training under my belt. Now I was older, bigger, leaner and a little smarter, I began to compare myself to physiques of professionals. I remember studying the muscles of one of the front cover models and being dismayed that he looked average. I was soon comparing my own physique to a professional, and that was the first time I thought maybe that could be me. The only difference between the model and me was that he'd put himself out there, while I was a complete unknown without any professional photographs to submit.

I wish I had taken more progress photos along the way, but I was not keen on having my photo taken, plus I grew up in an era before smartphones. I was in my late 20s before I took the leap and booked my first professional photo shoot. I didn't feel particularly photogenic, but the photographer complimented me greatly on my physique and asked if I'd ever considered competing on the stage. This wasn't something I'd thought about before, but I was certainly intrigued. It was a huge compliment. I decided to research some bodybuilding competitions. I'd seen some Mr Olympia tapes and it was clear the top guys were all taking steroids and I noticed the extreme size difference between myself and seasoned competitors from regional shows, as well. I realized I didn't stand a chance against professionals unless I started taking synthetics, but this was not a route I wanted to go.

CORE PRINCIPLE 1

CHART YOUR PROGRESS

How will you know if you've made progress if you don't take pictures? In my view, progress photos are a must.

You may not feel like doing this when you begin your journey, but nothing beats having something to look back on once you start making progress. Reflecting on how you used to look and how far you have come can be a very powerful and encouraging tool. Many people are moved to make a change because they see a photograph of themselves and don't like what they see.

Images can be a far more powerful medium than a measurement or a number on a scale and if you keep a log and take regular update photographs, this will inspire you to keep going.

The photographer I worked with told me there were natural (i.e. no performance-enhancing drugs) shows (see Resources for some examples) I could compete in, instead. After my photo shoot, I did a little research and registered with an agency. Initially, I was merely looking for somewhere to send my photos but then I noticed an advert for Mr UK – a natural bodybuilding event that offered competitors the opportunity to feature in a magazine.

In hindsight, it was more of a male beauty pageant than a bodybuilding competition, but I decided to go for it. I wanted to experience being up on a stage in front of an audience. It all seemed so glamorous, and a million miles away from the streets of North London where I'd grown up.

THE IMPORTANCE OF MENTORS

I've met many selfless people along the way who have had a lasting impact upon my life and career. Men like Fivos Averkiou, another athlete sponsored by PHD who selflessly helped me with nutrition and posing. I needed a lot of help with my diet, which I thought was okay at the time, but Fivos taught me about carb cycling and I am forever grateful for his advice.

Tim Gray – a fellow biohacker – opened man doors and connected me to so many people within the industry. I cannot stress enough the importance of surrounding yourself with positive role models.

Stepping out of my comfort zone

I was 31 years old when I first stepped onto the stage. I was sincerely petrified at the thought of getting up in front of an audience, and this made me feel I needed to do it even more.

As the show approached, I turned to my friends and family, trying to drum up some support. I told them this was my first competition and it would mean a lot to me if they could come along so there would at least be people I knew to cheer me on. They were excited for me and everyone promised to come but, as the day approached, my guests began to drop out one by one, until eventually nobody could make it. This made me even more nervous than I already was. Not only was I an introvert about to step on stage wearing close to nothing, but I had nobody coming to encourage me, either. I was all alone.

As I registered, I saw all of the other competitors and it slowly dawned on me that I would actually be competing on a stage in front of hundreds of spectators. Against men who might actually beat me. I was nervous talking to strangers, let alone standing on stage in front of judges to be studied and critiqued. All I wanted was a title, but when I started looking around, I noticed lots of younger guys with blue eyes and long blonde hair, some as young as 18 years old. More doubts crept in.

I seriously began to question what I had signed up for and why? Maybe it was a bad idea and there was still time to back out. I have a tendency to be quite instinctive when it comes to things like this. Spontaneous even. From experience, I knew if I thought too much about it, I would talk myself out of the situation. So, instead I held strong. I decided I needed to do this – to prove to myself that at least I had tried, regardless of the result.

Finally, we were called out in groups of four. We all stepped up to the T-walk in sequential order and it was there that the reality of the situation really hit me. I soon noticed that my competitors all had family and friends cheering them on, and here I was, and I didn't know a soul. What on earth was I doing? At that moment I felt like I'd entered a popularity contest with not a friend in the world.

As my turn came to go up, I nervously approached the stage. After watching the other competitors receive so much fanfare and encouragement from their friends and family – what seemed like the entire crowd cheering them on, blasting horns and blowing whistles and clapping fiercely – I walked out onto the catwalk to tumbleweed.

I stood in front of the crowd confronted by a deafening silence, and the only thing I could hear was the thumping sound from my own heart beating. At this point I felt terrible, self-doubt started to flow through my veins. I felt like an imposter. A fraud. But I couldn't back out now. I had to grin and bear it. So I did, with a smile on my face that was so fake I was sure everyone could see right through me.

I went through three rounds of this. In the first, we had to wear a suit. To make matters even more uncomfortable, I'd forgotten my tie, my belt and my socks. Still, I carried on. After a round in casual clothes, came the beachwear round. Now dressed in swimwear, it felt as if I was the only person not getting cheered. Again, I began to seriously doubt myself, wondering why I'd even bothered, but I persevered.

Eventually, it came to the placings at the end. All of the competitors were standing on the stage and when the presenter called out third place, I felt devastated that my name wasn't called, figuring I'd never place higher than that. Then, they called second and, of course, someone else's name was again called. I was sure that was that. I would smile and put on a brave face, like I had for much of the competition, and then I'd cheer for the winner and be a good sport.

Then, the announcer got ready to call the winner and he began dragging out the announcement, trying to increase the suspense. Eventually, they called out a name and I started to clap and smile; I tried to maintain some level of dignity, and I had so much doubt that I didn't even realize that the name that had been called was my own!

Everyone was looking around, trying to figure out what was going on and it wasn't until someone turned to me and said, "Aren't you Roger Snipes?" that it finally sank in. I'd won. I couldn't believe it. I almost cried. It wasn't just a case of winning; it was a really big deal for me. As a child I had been full of doubt and insecurity – this was finally the validation I had been searching for.

I had mixed emotions as I walked up to collect the trophy. *My* trophy. I was surprised, excited, humbled and triumphant. It felt so great. I didn't need anybody there to cheer me on; I had achieved this through my own hard work.

What I really enjoyed about being on the stage was the opportunity it allowed for me to step out of my comfort space and test my insecurities. Each time I had walked onto that stage, my heart had been full of palpitations. But it slowly softened away as I stood there with my prize. I whispered to myself, "you've won!"

Next steps

I wanted to prove that my first win wasn't a fluke, so I entered another competition, which I also went on to win. Afterwards, one of the announcers, who was an ex-bodybuilder, approached me and said, "you have a phenomenal physique. You should stop playing around in these pageants and enter an actual bodybuilding competition. That's where you'll really grow. That's where you'll be tested."

I didn't need any more encouragement than that. So, I went off and did a little more research and found a natural bodybuilding show called Musclemania, which I then went on to win.

I was sharing images on Facebook and was approached by a supplement brand who asked if I'd like to be sponsored by them. I remember thinking, this is it – I've made it! Free supplements, sponsorship from a known UK brand. Of course, I jumped at the chance. They invited me to an Expo called Body Power and suddenly I was being approached by delegates asking to have their photograph taken with me.

Being a sponsored athlete brought new pressures. I felt as though I needed to prove my worth, so I entered another competition – this time as a middleweight weighing 82kg (180lb) – and, to my astonishment, I won that also. It was amazing. I was winning shows. Random people wanted their photos taken with me. Then, I was contacted by ITV who wanted me to go on one of their shows to model underwear. An article about me ran in *Fabulous* magazine

(*News of the World*). Suddenly, I began getting loads of random friend requests on Facebook.

At this time, in the infancy of social media, I was a little perturbed; I was getting messages from strangers who had read the article or who had seen me on the television, and I found this quite unnerving. Friends of mine began joking, "You're famous now – these are your fans." I was actually messaging these people and asking why they were contacting me, and they told me they'd seen me in a magazine, or on the television. I felt like people were invading my private space. Fans? I really didn't get it; I was a nobody. But, eventually, I began to embrace the recognition, realizing I could use this platform to share my fitness journey. I began sharing more images and accepting friend requests, and that was the beginning of the training tips and videos that I now post regularly.

I competed in various shows until 2015, by which time I felt I had accomplished all I needed to. It was confidence that I was searching for, more than the trophies, although I do have these sitting in my office at home. To me, they symbolize courage. When I look at them it reminds me of how brave I was when it would have been so much easier to back out or quit.

So, seven shows, one sponsorship deal, a change of job and several magazine features later, I realized it wasn't beginner's luck after all. I didn't actually get on the front cover that had started this whole journey, but it didn't really matter. I still got all the validation I needed. I was finally putting my passion for fitness to some use and I'd found the focus I needed to take me to the next step.

ALWAYS GOING FORWARD

The Bible says, "Seek and you shall find. Ask and it shall be given to you. Knock on the door and it shall be opened to you". These profound words have always stuck with me and served me well to this day.

I remember being in my 20s and speaking with a 40-year-old man. He told me when I reached his age it would all go downhill, because of health and other issues. Twenty years later and my health has actually improved because I've had so many additional years of mental improvement. By investing so much in all areas of my health, I feel I've invested in my future, as well. Now, when I look in the mirror, I see a man in his 40s who is in the best mental and physical shape of his life. I still can't believe it, if I'm honest.

The important thing is to show up. Push yourself to get to the gym, then push yourself in the gym. Begin slowly, then build upon it and build upon it some more. Persevere. And always evaluate what works for you, and why.

DO YOUR RESEARCH

Today, I am as equally inspired by doctors and scientists as I once was with athletes and bodybuilders. These men and women on the forefront of genetic innovation have dedicated their lives to the improvement of the human being as a biological machine. People such as Dr Josh Axe, Dave Asprey, Dr Joseph Mercola, Ben Greenfield and Dr Steven R Gundry have further inspired my interest in genetic potential.

Discovering the research of these pioneers has allowed me to identify key areas that I have since sought to improve upon in my own training. I began to develop a great interest in dissecting the very act of exercise, of wellbeing and nutrition, in order to better understand the mechanics of my own body and the psychology of peak performance. After all, the vast majority of us are born with the same capabilities, and, health issues aside, the one thing that inhibits us is mindset.

SOCIAL MEDIA

I started to use social media around 2012. Like most people at the time, I used Facebook purely as a way to connect with family and close friends. It wasn't until later that I moved over to Instagram, where I began to share images and workout tips with an audience of relative strangers.

Instagram was slow to begin with. As my follower numbers rose, companies began to contact me, asking me to advertise their products. Brands began sending me free stuff with the caveat that I would promote their "gifts". I received everything from protein crisps to electronic scales. I started doing a lot of promotional stuff at the beginning, along with lots of daily posts, but as my platform grew, I began to get pickier with the products I wanted to promote, working with just a few reputable brands. This enabled me to work with companies that I admired, narrowing my focus and using my platform to build integrity.

Now I have over 750K followers on Instagram. Being on stage and front and centre definitely helped with my confidence, especially when posing and attending shoots. During my teenage years I hated having my photo taken and as a result there are very few pictures of me from back then. I was such an introvert. I hated smiling. But, being on the stage, almost naked in front of a crowd, really brought me out of my shell!

I think it's important to note that social media is not real. This is where people are presented at their best (and sometimes worst). A large following has nothing to do with your worth. While social media has its benefits, it's also important to detox and step away from it from time to time (*see* page 68).

MENTAL HEALTH

Mental Health is still a serious issue and is particularly prevalent in the age of social media, where status is measured by clicks and likes and blue ticks.

Men in particular are so afraid to show vulnerability in case it makes them appear weak, when in fact, the complete opposite is true. Accepting weakness can take a lot of courage, and it can also help you to improve.

Growing up, I was as an introvert. I was failing in school, while at home my weaknesses were consistently highlighted by my dad. This would of course upset me, which in turn further frustrated him. He was a man's man and I was taught that men do not show their feelings. Instead, he tried to instil strength in me, telling me that it was not manly to show weakness.

Even later on, when I began competing, my dad was un-supportive, making it clear he would have preferred that I'd chosen academics over aesthetics. Bearing in mind, my dad spent time in prison and was by no means a success himself, or any kind of role model. Clearly he was projecting his own feelings of failure and inadequacy onto me. Something that took me a long time to come to terms with.

In life, many people would rather put you down than support you. I knew I couldn't control my surroundings or the negative influences in my life, but I realized I could control my physique, and you can too. What I put into my body, and how I make it perform allow me to take control. These are the key things that continue to drive me.

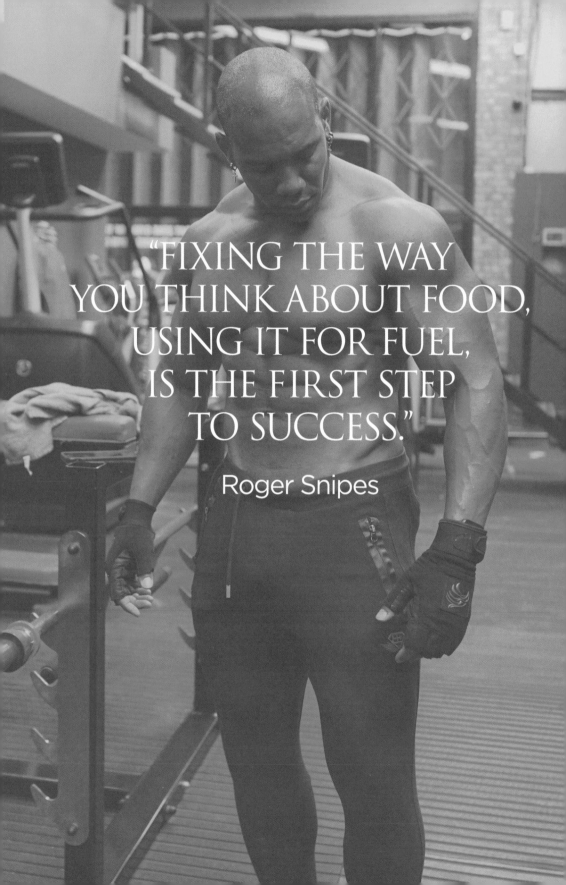

"FIXING THE WAY YOU THINK ABOUT FOOD, USING IT FOR FUEL, IS THE FIRST STEP TO SUCCESS."

Roger Snipes

CHAPTER 2
MIND OVER MATTER

The road to peak fitness begins with our human capacity for learning and knowledge. So, rather than dive into a training schedule without first considering what we are actually doing and why, I want us to take a moment to appreciate the one body part that we all seem to neglect The organ that decides everything.

I'm talking about the brain, of course. The organ that controls both hormones and muscle activity in the body. The brain also houses the mind, and this is responsible for our psychology and patterns of behaviour. The mind effectively drives the ship. It's responsible for choices and decision making and everything that we do.

While muscle mass combined with low body fat is usually the goal of most gym goers and fitness enthusiasts, this is also the result of a long-standing diet or training regime. However, the impetus of every training regime should begin firmly in the mind. I'm talking about visualisation. You've heard the term, "Mind over matter"? Well, this is where I want us to begin.

By exploring aspects of mindset and wellbeing before we hit the weights, I will aim to guide you along the rocky – and often vague – road of fitness and show you how best to prepare your brain and, therefore, your body for optimal enhancement. Bad habits are the things that inhibit us the most, so my aim is to give you strategies to deal with these before we move on to the weight rack. Cleansing the mind is where the real work begins.

Ultimately, the act of exercise and weight training is designed to inflict stress upon the body in order to make it respond and grow. The same way that stretching before a workout will better prepare your body, your mind needs to be readied in order to deal with the sudden change in activity and diet, and the recovery it will undergo. Throw yourself in at the deep end and try to do too much, too soon, and this will likely lead to failure or, worse still, giving up.

We will discover how the power of the mind can be harnessed to optimize your fitness experience in Part 2, but for now let's look at some of the basics.

The difference between exercise and bodybuilding

Exercise is part of "keeping fit". It's an activity, not necessarily an overhaul. Exercise doesn't concern itself primarily with the aesthetic: it's about staying active, feeling healthy, maintaining flexibility and, more often than not, it's about having fun.

Bodybuilding, on the other hand, is about looks, and is taken very seriously by practitioners. It involves hours of heavy weights and meal prep. It's where art meets science. It's a combination of sculpture and biology, where muscle mass, definition and vascularity are as important as attaining the lowest possible percentage of body fat.

This book is about both of these things, and more. It's about feeling good on the inside, while looking the best you can on the outside. This is a plan for total self-overhaul. It's the whole package. I want to explore overall physical and mental improvement, looking at fitness from all sides, exploring muscle growth while also providing some basic scientific knowledge. Remember we're looking at 100% steroid-free options, utilizing biohacking to tap into our own inner resources, unlocking your inner power naturally.

CORE PRINCIPLE 2

SEPARATE FACT FROM FICTION

There is a lot of misinformation within the fitness world. People often fail to take bodybuilding seriously as a sport because of controversies surrounding performance-enhancing drugs, or because bodybuilders are labelled as boneheads. In fact, bodybuilders have always been ahead of the curve where the latest trends in nutrition and fitness are concerned. While anabolic steroids (synthetic hormones) do aid weight loss, natural bodybuilders don't use them and have been following the principles of "clean eating" and the benefits of "whole foods" for many years (*see* page 110).

In recent years, we've seen ketogenic diets, clean eating and intermittent fasting become trends within the mainstream, but bodybuilders have been using these diet principles for decades, in order to get as lean as possible for the stage.

FACT: Some bodybuilders take steroids.

FICTION: All bodybuilders take steroids.

FACT: Bodybuilders were the first biohackers.

Bodybuilders have always used the basic principles of science to push the boundaries of human physicality. Granted, some have pushed it a little too far, but we should not discredit how pioneering the sport has been in terms of attaining peak physicality and human advancement.

So, do your research, don't jump to conclusions or subscribe to stereotypes, and be sure to separate fact from fiction. Give some of the latest innovations described in this book a chance. You might be surprised at what you learn.

What is health and how do we measure it?

It goes without saying that we should be utilizing every opportunity to harness the power of health to instil longevity of life. But, of course, spending all day in the gym or exercising is both impractical and impossible for all but the most elite athletes and gym professionals. Likewise, working with a nutritionist is beyond the budget of most people. We also have to contend with everything else life has to throw at us along the way – family, work, friends, socializing, shopping and entertainment, and so many other commitments.

I believe that those of us who are in good health should do everything we can to maintain it, and those who need improvement should live and breathe fitness to better themselves. Why? Because, first and foremost, basic fitness is free (or reasonably inexpensive). All it costs is time and effort, and maybe the investment of some basic kit. Working out for just a few days a week will greatly improve your life. Second, once your fitness has gone it's difficult to regain. As soon as you find yourself on the wrong side of unfit, the older you become, the more difficult you will find it to return to your best state. And When you reach middle age, this is where you're going to miss it the most.

Therefore, our physical (and mental) health, much like our diets, should always be central to our lives. These are fundamental to our wellbeing and should be as important, if not more so, than money or success. Many people dream of immortality, but don't want to put in a little bit of effort to prolong the time they've already got. It's so easy to neglect the assets we have and focus instead on material things, but you cannot buy good health and it's quite difficult to put a measure on it, as well. We know what "fit" looks like and what being fit feels like, but what does "healthy" actually look like?

THE MIND IS A MUSCLE

Like all muscles, the mind needs to be tested and trained.

It also needs to be rested.

Bad habits, cravings and poor diets are almost always part of one's own state of mind.

food is information which synergistically works with or against our biological functions. Fixing the way you think about it – using it for fuel rather than as an appetite suppressant, or eating to alleviate boredom or stress – is the first step to success.

Ask 100 people and you'll receive 100 different answers from: lean, fast, thin, muscular, curvaceous, glowing, bright-eyed, energetic, happy

So, is health merely a state of mind? Is poor health a matter of illness, or of complacency? Or perhaps both?

It's easy to judge how you look in the mirror, or what you weigh on the scale. But to get a balanced overall picture of one's health is quite difficult. What does a healthy lifestyle look like?

There is no one answer. Health relates to a number of combining factors. All of the things mentioned above and more. *Being* healthy and *looking* healthy are two different things. You might look fit, but real health comes from within – it is really a combination of knowledge, balance and self-care.

Be a constant work in progress

The one thing above all others that has inspired me to write this book is the one question I get asked more than any other, and it's the very same thing I've asked myself ever since I began lifting weights in my bedroom. It's this:

"How can I make my body perform better?"

I can't lie. The physique I have now took years of hard graft – and that's the one thing you need to be prepared for. This isn't a quick-fix 12-week programme, it's an overhaul meant for life. The moment you stop working out or eating well, your body will start to revert to the state it was when you began. Of course, you can take a break, or take days off, but improvement and sustaining fitness levels is a constant work in progress.

So, in order to maintain, or to improve, you will need to find space within the shape of your day to do some work. I am still learning, still looking to improve, and I still struggle to fit everything in. But I make the time, and quite often that requires sacrifices. If you want to change, then be prepared to adapt. Give up an hour of your day, even just a few times per week. You don't need to join a gym, but it has a lot of advantages. Without one you will be limited in what you can do, and the investment of joining a gym will also force you to work a lot harder.

No shortcuts

I've trained with some of the best in the business. I've also spent many years researching every fad, topic, innovation and advancement in the industry in my quest to better my knowledge and understanding of peak human experience. I have competed in bodybuilding shows, worked with experts in the field of scientific research, and travelled the world attending expos and trade shows, both as a guest speaker and also as a sponsored athlete. Every one of these things was possible because of the physique that I've built with my own two hands. My body, much like the information I am going to share with you in this book, has been a labour of love and my life's work. And all of this is built upon a strong mental foundation – a positive mindset that keeps me motivated and enjoying the life I choose to lead.

Before we move on to Part 2, I think it's important to recap some of the guiding principles of this book.

This is not a "journey" or a get fit quick scheme. There is no such thing as 'a perfect physique'. Look instead for peak health and fitness instead. Take a transformational approach which requires sustained dedication. There are plenty of tips and hacks that I can teach you, but there are *no shortcuts for peak fitness*.

The rules are incredibly simple: all it takes to build your perfect physique is willpower, determination, a set of self-imposed guidelines and a lot of hard, hard work. And, of course, perseverance. Do not rush. Don't cut corners. Take your time. Make an effort to soak up as much information as you can.

The reason 8- or 12-week programmes never work is because people fall off the wagon once they've seen some results, or they stop altogether. So, the sooner you think of this as your new lifestyle and not as a quick-fit programme, the better.

In essence, in this guide I aim to debunk myths and distinguish "bro science" from real scientific techniques, providing you with a fundamental framework and the confidence to tailor a programme to your individual needs. So take what you need.

Consider it a long, but worthwhile lifestyle change. In a few years' time, you'll thank past-you. That is a guarantee.

MIND OVER MATTER

Have daily rituals

How you begin your day can strongly determine how it ends. Every morning when I wake up, I follow a set of rules that help me get my mind in order. I think of them as mental housekeeping or emptying my brain's inbox. A strong mindset comes from uncluttered thoughts.

I reckon it's easy to look at me and think I must spend all day, every day in the gym, but I don't spend nearly as much time working out as you might think. I work out maybe two or three times a week with weights and will also try to factor in some time to get outside, whether that be to jog in the park, or to cycle.

A large proportion of my day is actually spent in front of my computer, either working on my business, posting on social media, or working on other investments that I have set up. It is essential, therefore, that I begin each day by following a simple structure, focusing first on myself, before I focus on anything outside.

Every single morning I practise some deep-breathing techniques, followed by a little red light therapy, using a red-light panel (*see* page 122). Red light can provide infrared and aid cellular health, but it does not supply vitamin D. If you are deficient in vitamin D you should consider a supplement (*see* page 121). The red light does help to promote collagen in skin, as well as healthy cartilage and joints. I will usually have a red light panel positioned directly in front of me that I switch on and off at 20-minute intervals – this helps to boost mitochondria, which aids protein synthesis. While I do all this, I will also be attached to a device called a Nano-V, which helps with cellular repair and daily oxidative stress, while also promoting anti-ageing. I will do all of this with my feet firmly on an earthing or grounding mat (*see* pages 120-21), which helps to protect me while using a laptop connected to WIFI, and while Electro-magnetic Frequencies (EMFs) are emitted. Read more about my daily biohacks in Part 3.

However well you map things out, your life will have a way to shake that up. Lack of time, or everyday obstacles will be thrown your way, and people often then use this as an excuse to skip the workout or eat unhealthy food. "I don't have the time." We've all said it. But you can gain control by having a bit of structure in place in your day, starting off first thing, and this will then become the norm, provided you enforce it.

If I'm away travelling, I'll instead use whatever natural methods are available to me in terms of boosting energy and longevity. I'll walk barefoot outside, expose my skin to natural light, take deep breaths of fresh air. I'll stretch. The reason we generally feel so relaxed when we're on holiday is because we find ourselves closer to nature. For example, we tend to expose more skin or walk barefoot on the beach.

Whenever you get an opportunity, I recommend you try walking or jogging barefoot on the grass or meditating out in the open.

Spending so much time indoors, and in front of a screen, is not ideal for health or wellbeing. I try to counter this as much as I can by getting outside in natural daylight, where possible. Too much exposure to blue light from screens can affect your circadian rhythm and your ability to sleep, so when I am forced to stay in, to combat any potential ill effects I will also wear blue-light blocker glasses if I'm sitting in front of a computer screen for long periods of time.

Another of my morning rituals is to check in with my goals for that year, and to practise gratitude. This reminds me of the things I am grateful for; things that I have accomplished in my life, where I have come from and how far I have come. It enables me to get some perspective and is a good counterbalance to my striving for goals I have not yet achieved. I cover goals and gratitude in greater detail on pages 63–4.

MIND OVER MATTER

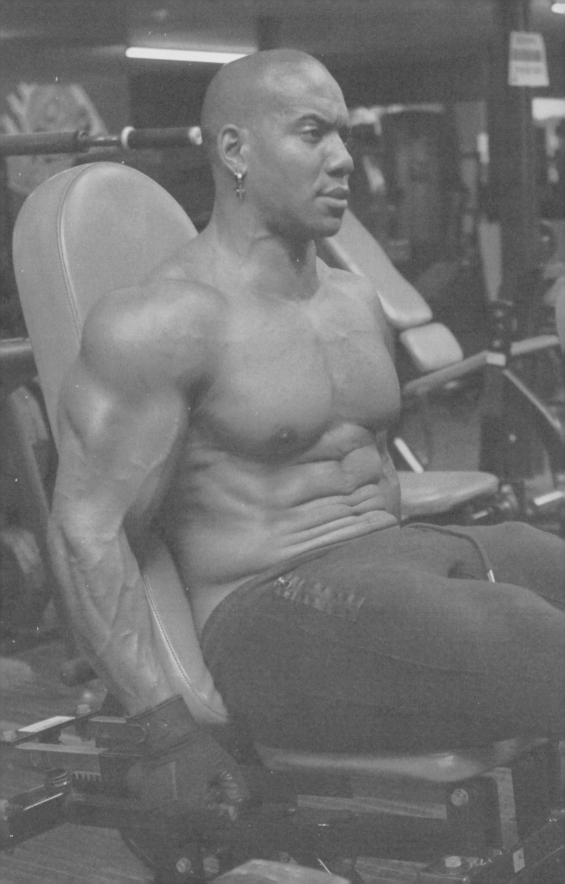

PART 2

Use the Power of the Mind

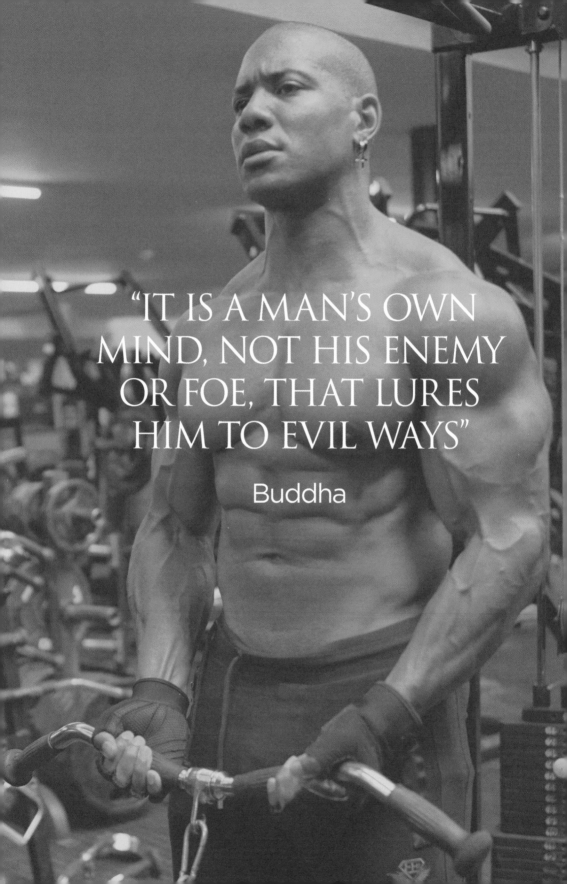

"IT IS A MAN'S OWN
MIND, NOT HIS ENEMY
OR FOE, THAT LURES
HIM TO EVIL WAYS"

Buddha

CHAPTER 3

GET YOUR MIND ON BOARD

More often than not, failure translates into two words: "I can't."
"I can't be bothered. I can't find the time. I can't get motivated. I can't get to the gym."

If "I can't" is holding you back, perhaps your mind is not in the right place, or maybe you're housing emotional baggage that needs shifting before you begin. If you have a mental block, are too busy, or too tired, then you are going to struggle to reach, but more importantly, maintain your goals. These things need to be addressed or they will forever be a burden.

This chapter will look at some of the tools and tricks I have used over the years to enable me to overcome mental obstacles in order to develop a physique that has, in turn, helped me become a success in the fitness industry and bodybuilding world.

Fitness is a feat of the mind

Fitness is a process of learned behaviours. It's where psychology meets physiology, simple as that. Just think, your mind can raise or lower your heart rate. It can improve or interfere with your digestion through stress, and it can change the chemical composition of your blood. It can help or hinder your sleep. It can also create psychological limitations, taking us back to those dreaded words, "I can't".

We want to be coming from a place of confidence, developing good mental habits that build resilience and positivity, taking you anywhere you want to go in terms of your fitness goals.

You see, with confidence comes a heightened sense of self-assurance. It's that moment when you *know* you can hit a certain weight, or attain a certain body-fat percentage, and then the act itself becomes a matter of fact.

Nobody walks into the gym thinking they can bench-press 80kg (177lb). But as soon as you hit that target, it will forever remain an "I CAN" in your mind. It's just like riding a bike. You, and your body, won't forget you can do it.

Retrain the brain

Fitness is all about hurdles and hard work and pushing yourself beyond what you're used to. You will need to work extra hard to instil patience and build resilience in order to meet the many challenges you are likely to face. But most of these challenges will be your mind telling you this is new and therefore not what you're used to.

You know the feeling: that slump you get whenever you've been out of the gym for an extended period of time, or the slog you feel when you force your way through a run or a workout when you're not feeling up to it. Your body just won't stop complaining. The pain, the dread, the exhaustion and then the added failure of feeling unfit; it's all enough to make you give in before you've even begun.

If you've had days, weeks, or even years of not exercising, feeling unfit or too tired to train, getting started can feel like a real mountain to climb. This first hurdle is where most people fail before they've even begun. But if you start with a little work on your mind, you will be able to take these crucial first steps.

Set your intention to transform your health and life. Think about your goals and write down some first small steps to get you started. Daily rituals, as explained in the previous chapter, can really help to get you focused and keep you on the right track.

As I've already said, patience is key. And resilience, too. You will need to build up to tackling your goals.

This will all help to train your mind to forge new habits, and soon enough you will begin to FEEL the benefits, even before you SEE them. This is very important to remember. Instilling good diet and training practices will make your body function more efficiently; you will feel better inside – giving you more energy, more vitality, more impetus to train – and the outside, visible results will follow.

And the process is cyclical. You just have to make sure that your behaviour is following an upward, not downward, spiral. For example, the more junk you eat, the less energy you'll have, and the less likely you'll want to work out. This makes you more likely to feel low, making it more likely you will eat junk to make you feel better, and so on.

On the other hand, the more you train, and the more you eat right, the better you will feel inside. This will propel you to work out more and it will most likely deter you from eating that big greasy meal, or having too much sugar, which will lead to continuing improvements in your diet, which makes you feel better.

Take baby steps

Your mind will give in to temptation long before your body does, which is why practising resilience is so important. That desire to succeed comes from within. Your body is the RESULT of good (or bad) choices. If you do not have a firm resolve before you even begin, then there is your problem. The main obstacle hindering you starting to exercise / eat well is in your mind. Thankfully, the mind can be conditioned the same way you can condition a muscle, and that is done through simple ritual and routine.

Conditioning yourself to live a healthy lifestyle is best done in stages.

If your body is not conditioned to lift heavy weights yet, or you haven't built up a resilience to working out four or five days a week, then ease yourself into it.

If you don't, it's likely that you'll suffer from Delayed Onset Muscle Soreness (DOMS), or worse still, injury. Start with lighter weights and training once or twice a week. Eventually, your body will tell you that more is okay.

The same principle goes for your diet. If you've been overeating or indulging in junk food for an extended period of time, and then you quickly transition into a low-carb, no-sugar diet, or you move straight onto a ketogenic diet or intermittent fasting (*see* p93-8), your body will reject this. You'll suffer headaches or hunger pangs and it's likely you'll crash. And crashing will send you on a fast track straight back to junk food with your mind translating everything you've tried to do as an impossible task that you would rather avoid.

Follow good habits

Those who fail where fitness is concerned usually do so because they approach it in one of two ways. Either they look at exercise as a chore, thereby resenting every minute of it, or they become so desperate for results that they either burn out too quickly or give up because the results aren't coming fast enough.

Remember: nobody gets out of shape overnight.

USE THE POWER OF THE MIND

Being overweight or unfit will be the culmination of weeks, months or maybe years of following the same bad habits. Likewise, reversing those bad habits will take time. The very word "routine" translates as "path" or "course".

Habits, too, take time to correct – they require an understanding of physiology to steer you along the right path; they require mental strength in order to stay on course. So, before you can break through that mental barrier you need to be fully prepared upstairs.

The right approach

Humans thrive on autopilot – this is our safe spot, our comfort zone. The mind and body work in tangent and both will revert to the path of least resistance in order to preserve the status quo. As such, your immediate needs will always supersede your long-term goals.

The key to long-term fitness is habit. I can't emphasize this enough. When we form long-lasting habits, our minds and bodies will adapt to this new way of doing things. Our muscles develop memory and in no time at all, following our new plan becomes second nature.

There is no secret trick or magic hack to get around this. You just need to work harder and smarter, and be consistent in what you do. Effectively, you need to realign your body with healthier behaviours.

You can start creating these healthier behaviours straight away. Begin by cutting out a certain food group – something like bread or sweets – and take it from there. Add a free-weight workout once a week to your routine. Get a smartwatch, Fitbit or use the health tracker app on your phone to count how many steps you take each day, and then challenge yourself to beat that week's total.

Up your work rate a step at a time and this will soon add up.

CORE PRINCIPLE 3

LOOK AT THE BIGGER PICTURE

When embarking on a new path in life, a little perspective is essential. If you focus solely on the problem, you may never see the solution, as simple as it might be.

Before zoning in and breaking down your new workout schedule or eating plan, make sure you have already taken a look at the bigger picture. If your aim is to get a flat stomach, or more muscular arms, or to increase your bench press, take some steps back to work out what you need to do to achieve this. Focusing on the subcutaneous fat around your middle will not help you lose it, neither will doing 800 sit-ups. You cannot spot-reduce fat. Your focus should instead be on lowering your overall body-fat percentage, and you will achieve this by moving more and eating less. It's that simple. A good diet will improve your six-pack more than sit ups ever will.

Likewise, to improve your biceps, you should focus on compound lifts to strengthen skeletal muscles and overall strength. Work your triceps just as hard. They are twice as big after all, and will make your arms look much bigger. The biceps will come as a result of working out your entire upper body, rather than just doing curls all day.

Know what you are working toward. Give yourself a clear overall goal, and really consider what you need to do and how far you have to go to get there. Make a list of everything you want to achieve and write it down. Then construct your own programme, keep a log of your development, keep taking those progress photos, and you'll soon be achieving your goals.

You are what you do

The idea of physical perfection is a matter of opinion and this is, of course, relative to one's own idea of the perfect physique. For some, that will be based on pure size, while for others, the ideal might be determined by function.

For example, a sprinter will look quite different to a long-distance runner or a swimmer. Each will develop a body shape based upon their unique training programmes and sport-specific diets. Training for these sports will focus on certain exercises specific to that activity to enable the athlete to enhance the relevant muscle groups.

Swimmers may not necessarily train their traps and lat muscles for size, but these muscle groups will still grow naturally and disproportionately from other, less utilized muscles, because of the repetition of certain actions during their training. This happens because of a combination of nature and necessity: the repetitive nature of the exercise, and the excessive constant tension they are put under. The body's need to perform certain functions grows through adaptation, the same way a swimmer's lung capacity will also become greater over time, because it needs to hold onto air for long periods of time. Sprinters, meanwhile, will usually be muscular with larger quad muscles and upper body strength, while long-distance runners will be much leaner, despite the sports being of similar disciplines. Their muscles form out of necessity and through repetition. The body learns, and then it adapts.

This is how our minds develop, too. If fitness and health become part of who you are, you are more likely to become conditioned over time. For example, if you go a prolonged period of time without eating sugar, then eating something sugary will create an insulin spike / sugar rush that will, in turn, cause you to crash. Crashing will make you feel tired, thus, leaving you with a perceived lack of motivation.

However, what you perceive as a lack of motivation is more likely a weak mindset, and this is what's really sabotaging your progress. This is how your body has been conditioned. You want a flat stomach for your holiday in six weeks, but you want a biscuit right now. The biscuit will probably win if you only plan for today.

GETTING STARTED

Here are some top tips and hacks that will help you get a good start on your fitness journey:

›› Buy clean food
›› Introduce activity into your day
›› Train on a regular basis
›› Educate yourself – read health books and listen to health podcasts
›› Follow inspirational people on social media
›› Focus on building healthy relationships
›› Get the family involved: introduce them to whole foods and exercise
›› Use healthy affirmations
›› Visualize being healthy

When your whole life is saturated with health-related stuff, it soon becomes second nature. You can't fail because this is all you know, and soon enough you'll want to be the best you can be, because a healthy mentality is addictive.

You are also what you don't do

Your body is ultimately the by-product of routine and will reflect what you do every day. This is why banishing bad habits and forming a positive mindset is essential to your health.

If you sit at a desk all day, for years on end, fat will eventually begin to store in pockets around your seat area: bottom, waist and hips. Conversely, if you spend enough of the day, every day, on the move, the chances are your physique will reflect this. Big changes come about as a result of lots of small incremental everyday things and not just one alteration. Changing your diet while remaining sedentary will have little effect. You will be spinning the wheels if you work out like a maniac and then eat chocolate or drink beer as a treat for all of your hard work. You can't outwork a bad diet. The negative will always counter the positive.

Willpower comes first. Build this and banish weakness of mind and your health will benefit. Fitness is health and health should come before everything, because without it, nothing else exists.

If you base your daily routine around things that improve your health and fitness, you will soon find it difficult to live any other way. However, if you base your fitness goals around everything else in your life, you may well struggle to fit it in and fall victim to one of the biggest obstacles of all: making excuses. Here's a list of some of the most common excuses I hear:

>> **I work long hours**
>> **I'm tired after work**
>> **I have children**
>> **I'm married**
>> **I work shifts**
>> **It's too cold**
>> **It's too hot**

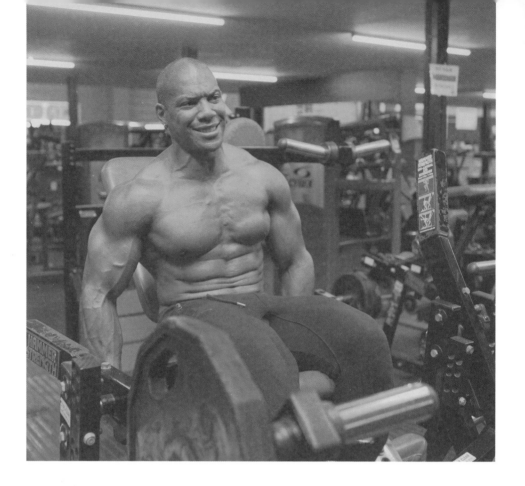

Put your fitness goals at the top of your list. Being fitter and building strength will give you more energy to be your best in all of the other areas of your life, too. It's a no-brainer, if you ask me. And always make sure you have a contingency plan – for example, have a shorter home workout up your sleeve if an unforeseen event means you genuinely can't get to the gym that day.

On those days where you feel you're too tired or can't face a gym visit: commit to doing 5 minutes of movement at home. Chances are, 5 minutes will energize you and lead to you doing more. And if you're genuinely tired, maybe 5 minutes will be enough to help you sleep well and recover stronger. Don't allow your mind to sabotage what your body needs.

USE THE POWER OF THE MIND

CHAPTER 4

DO A SELF-APPRAISAL

In our fast-paced society, we tend to make conscious decisions that limit our focus to only the things we deem truly worthy of our attention and energy. Whether that is work or education, or our private lives, we narrow in and tend to ignore things that we see as not vital. And sometimes our health and wellbeing can end up being little more than an afterthought as a result.

Self-development creates self-awareness. When you strive to better yourself, when you show love to yourself and have full respect for the person you see in the mirror, then you'll make better selections. So, in this chapter, we'll take a good look at ourselves, what makes us tick, and how we can support our minds to be a solid foundation from where we can achieve our goals.

Identity: understand your DNA

WHO ARE YOU, REALLY?

A loss or lack of identity is one of the key issues faced by modern humans. It's hard to know who we are at the core when so many of our behaviours have been accumulated from our ancestors, families and our peers. Many of us suffer from imposter syndrome too, or low self esteem, without considering how we ended up the way we are.

But how we view ourselves, and how we think others see us can truly affect our approach to life. The act of self-analysis (which is more often than not a reflection of how we think others perceive us) can make us feel powerful, but it can also make us feel powerless, if we think others see us in a bad light.

So, get to know yourself. Not who you want to be, or what you want to look like, but who you are right now. Take time out and look in the mirror. If there are things you do that are detrimental to your wellbeing, ask yourself "Why?" Be accountable. Are they learned behaviours, things that have been ingrained since childhood? Are they embedded within your DNA?

It is paramount that we understand who we are and why we make the choices that we do in order to make progress and better ourselves. However, we shouldn't dwell on the things we don't like, especially around appearance and physique. Not liking what you see can lead to detrimental behaviours and even self-loathing, so remember that some things are just down to genetics – you have to work with what you've got, rather than wish you were different. Wishing isn't going to change anything.

Instead, admit you could make improvements and then strive to work harder on those problem areas. (This is why progress pictures are so important.) Identify the key areas that need work, but don't forget to take note of the areas and things that you like about yourself, as well.

Rewire inherited traits

There is no denying, genetics do play a major part in one's body composition – but they also determine behaviours and habits as well. The good news is that our brains are constantly forming new connections and pathways, and it is possible to build new habits and behaviours through repetition.

But let's get back to your body. If your dad is muscular, chances are you will be too. Or you will at least have the same genetic propensity. Unfortunately, stress and obesity are also genetic traits; there is just no getting around that. While many men and woman struggle to keep weight off, others may fight to put on mass. For example, certain body types will struggle with leg size, or abdominal definition. The point is, your genetics are pre-determined, so forget about what you don't have and work to make what you've got as good as it can be.

Regardless of genetics, willpower, focus and drive will always beat a good base. You can always improve upon your natural state. You may need to make more sacrifices, or work harder, because of your genetic makeup, but doing nothing and allowing nature to take its course will ultimately take you back to square one.

Get out of autopilot

Exercise alone is not enough. Don't just think about training, but try to consider the everyday logistics of health, as well. Adapt the things you do without thinking, and try to incorporate incremental changes into your everyday routine.

For example, if you walk to work, take a slightly longer route. Get your step count up. Log your progress. Get off the bus a couple of stops early. Take a little time to read labels on the food you buy and figure out what exactly is in the things you are consuming – especially hidden sugars. All of these things add up, whether it's an extra few steps or a little less sugar. By adapting your everyday routine, you can begin to lay the foundations for a brand new you.

Routine versus structure versus ritual

In essence, these three words mean the same thing, but just by re-framing the way we think about how we live our lives can give meaning to the things we do. Routines conjure a sense of boredom because routines can become stale over time. Structures, likewise, are rigid. Rituals, on the other hand, invoke a sense of ceremony and reward.

DO A SELF-APPRAISAL

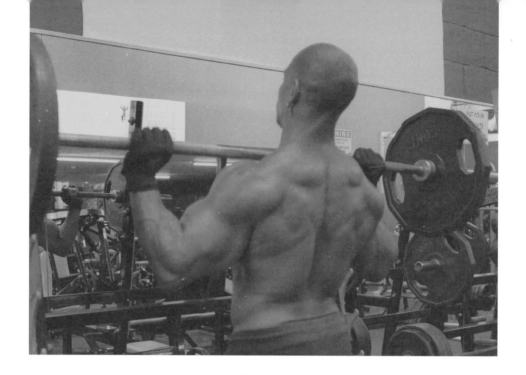

Humans covet structure. Maybe this is passed down from our ancestors. It's in our DNA. Venturing outside the parameters of our natural habitat feels instantly uncomfortable. But, of course, we don't grow as people if we don't push boundaries.

Whether that's going to a fitness class for the first time, or adapting to a new diet (after all, most of the bad foods we eat are of course comfort foods), we instantly look to something easy and familiar when we are feeling low or lacking energy.

So, if you want to change, don't settle for "easy".

Make a plan. Add something new to your daily routine. Then map out what you need to do and do your best to stick to it.

A little planning will go a long way and will add structure and routine to your life.

CORE PRINCIPLE 4

DEFINE YOUR OWN STRATEGY

Fitness is about detail. It's about variables. It's the combining of factors; creating the right environment in order to aid change. It's about adopting a strategy that works for you. While diet alone (being in a calorie deficit) will help you lose weight, combining the right meal plan with exercise will help accelerate weight loss further. Likewise, lifting heavy weights while eating in a calorific surplus should build muscle (but perhaps some fat, also). It will certainly help you gain size.

There is so much to know. There are so many options, routes, and opinions to consider. For example:

>> What is the best pre-workout, post-workout, mid-workout energy boost?
>> Should I do cardio or weights or both?
>> Should I train fast or full?

There is no right or wrong answer because everyone is different. It's easy for us fitness types to lecture because fitness is our job. That's why the most valuable advice I can give you is this: be open to trying new things. Pick a diet and exercise programme that is slightly outside of your comfort zone to begin with, and then push yourself a little harder each week. Remember, baby steps.

Create your own strategies and write them down. This way you have something to check back on. It's important that your progress is measurable. You will become better, faster, leaner, stronger, so make sure you move the goalposts a little bit at a time, in order to challenge yourself without creating an impossible task. Soon enough, your end goal will become the starting point for your next challenge.

Engage your brain 🎙

Preparing your mind for battle is, in many ways, like rehabbing an injury. You have to ease into it and gradually build up your strength and resilience, rather than steaming in, all guns blazing, and giving yourself DOMS. And don't half-arse your workout – spinning the wheels – then become frustrated because you look the same as you did six months ago. The worst thing you can do in the gym is go through the motions. If your body is doing the work while your mind is absent from the process, chances are, you're not putting enough effort in. An engaging workout will require you to think about what you are doing. If you're lifting heavy weights then it's imperative that you be switched on, in order to both engage and stay safe.

So, when prepping for a new workout – whether that be leg day, or an upper body / lower body split, or even some High Intensity Interval Training (HIIT) – take some time to work on what's inside and that will help you on your way. We tend to spend plenty of time thinking about hitting our reps and sets and making our macros fit a daily allowance, but forget to check in with our head to see if it's in a good place.

When approaching a workout, let your mind warm up a little before you begin. Make sure that you're in the right headspace. Introduce some rituals – breathing, meditation, gratitude lists, a morning grounding practice (*see* pages 120-1) – into your daily routine that let you focus on harnessing your mental energy. I guarantee this will improve your workout and the way you view training. Feeling better on the inside is the first step to looking better on the outside.

Take a moment every morning for yourself. Spend some time meditating or focusing on what you want to achieve. Check in with your goals – short, medium and long-term – and think about what you need to do to take a step closer to them. Make a note of your strengths, as well, and be grateful for them. We all strive to be better, but need to frame things positively.

USE THE POWER OF THE MIND

Practising gratitude (*see* pages 63-6). Set aside some thinking time like this gives you a chance to consider what you want to achieve and how you can get there. Is the target realistic? If so, set clear achievable goals that are both practical and measurable.

Everyone who ever joined a gym or picked up a book like this is looking for a way to improve themselves. That goes without saying. But I want you to think about what you're doing both in *and* out of the gym with a view to help you overhaul everything.

Success is something earned. Once in a blue moon, an individual or a team may achieve success through sheer luck, but continued success requires strategy and hard work.

Bad habits are driven by the mind, so in order to overcome these and see results, create a plan that works for you. The worst thing you can do is force yourself to join a gym or begin a diet that makes you to reach too hard and too fast. This isn't a race, so take your time and use your brain to create your own bespoke strategy.

MAKE THE CONNECTION
I cannot stress how important the mind-muscle connection is.

The next time you work out a body part, try to really focus on the actual muscle that you're hitting, rather than just the weight you're lifting or the repetition.

You should feel the muscle contract as you place it under stress and then the pump afterwards as blood fills the muscle.

DO A SELF-APPRAISAL

Motivation alone is not enough

People often talk about incentives, or what motivates them, but I think the word "motivation" is overused to the point where it's virtually meaningless.

To me, motivations are shallow. They usually come from an external source – maybe a poster or a quote – and are something we use to fuel us for a short time. A song can motivate you to run faster, or to lift heavier ... for a short period of time.

Motivation is like sugar. It's a spark, or a quick fix remedy, but motivation alone is not enough when you're feeling hungry or tired, or stuck, or ready to give in. I also liken it to an ejector seat: it'll get you off your backside fast, but pretty soon you'll come crashing back down to where you began.

If you expect to stay motivated all day every day because you read an inspirational quote or saw a photo of someone you want to look like, then you'll need to seek that out every single day. That's like asking the sun to shine for a specific amount of time and to the right degree. It's like expecting canaries to sing to you every morning by your bedside window, just so you can wake up happy.

It's asking for conditions to be *just right*.

If you have to try to constantly find that spark to urge you on, then you're going to burn yourself out before you've begun. You're going to need something far more fundamental and longer-lasting than this ...

What you need to build is a strong, well-fuelled internal drive.

Drive is key

Looking at a photograph of a nice house might seem like motivation enough to get rich. But it's not going to make you rich. You get rich either by luck or because you have the type of internal drive that won't let you quit until you've reached your goal.

Likewise, you don't work out because you read a quote on Instagram, regardless of how much it might have chimed with you at the time. You work out and eat right because you genuinely want to be in the best physical shape you can be.

That's not to say you won't look at a photograph of Arnold Schwarzenegger in his prime and think, I want to look like that. But you can't rely on that as motivation alone, unless you're going to whip it out every time you fancy a biscuit. It's not enough.

Sometimes, these things we consider "motivational" actually have the opposite effect, because we realize we may never buy that big house, or look like Arnold. What then?

Instead, use things that fuel your inner *drive* instead. Consider the things that get you excited for. Something you want so badly that you will not stop until it's yours. Envision your end goal. Drive and determination are the things that will push you through the tough times. These are the key ingredients for success. After all, "I am driven" is a lot more powerful than "I am motivated".

Drive is what really makes us get up in the morning. It challenges us; it makes us go to the gym, it makes us eat the right meals at the right times. It makes us strive for success. It is the culmination of habit and small incremental strategies that ultimately add up to the whole.

It is the embodiment of success.

DO A SELF-APPRAISAL

DON'T GET STUCK IN A RUT

Sometimes people will go to the gym and follow the same tired routine until they grow grey hairs.

And for some people this works. If you're gaining strength and / or size and that is your overall goal, then why change it? Stick with your routine and continue making results.

However, if you've read this far then chances are you're looking for change.

People go to the gym to train and get results, but they also go because the commitment of a gym contract forces them to work out. At least, that's the theory, but it can also begin to feel like a chore over time. It's like doing the same old job. Pretty soon the novelty wears off and you're looking for excuses not to go. That dread of getting there becomes another hump to get over. This is the stage where people begin to search for 'motivation' in order to keep going.

And as I've discussed:

›› If you need constant incentives, then you're going to encounter constant obstacles as well.

›› If your routine begins to feel mundane, or it is not paying off, then change it up. Train outside or at home if you can't face the gym. Split your workouts up with an activity or a sport.

And remember: It's not failure unless you continue doing something that doesn't work.

Give gratitude

With so much focus on strategies, goals and success, it's easy to lose sight of the things we already have that we are grateful for. A key part of my holistic approach to health and fitness – mental, physical and emotional – is practising gratitude.

Gratitude is an appreciation of the basic things that you have. The life you have. The food in your fridge. Your friends, colleagues and family.

I remember a time in my life when I had so much debt. I was in temporary accommodation that was infested with mice and I was sleeping on a mattress on the floor. Looking back at moments like that make me very grateful for what I have now.

Gratitude is a reminder of where we are and how far we have come. It enables us to appreciate everything that we have already achieved. It has also been shown to have many benefits for our mental and physical health. By just taking the time to remember a few things each day that you are grateful for you can expect to experience more positive emotions, get better sleep and even boost your immune system.

So write down what you are grateful for.

The moment your eyes open in the morning, it often feels like a starting gun has gone off and the race begins. You are bombarded with lists to run through and try to complete before your day is done. Rather than taking time to reflect we set up new things to do and proceed with the daily cycle.

That's why a Gratitude List (in my head or written down) is on my to-do list before anything else. Before reading emails, WhatsApp, texts, social media or logging onto the world, I confess my gratitude.

DO A SELF-APPRAISAL

Take a moment. Relax and appreciate your health. Even if it's not 100 percent If you have a home then you have shelter. Appreciate the basic stuff that you take for granted. It is important to feel grounded sometimes, especially when the world around you is travelling at a million miles per hour.

A Gratitude List will condition you to appreciate the small things in life, which are often the most important. If you don't want to do it at the beginning of the day, work out a good time for you. Sometimes last thing at night is the perfect time.

Learn from your mistakes

Learning from your own mistakes is good, but learning from the mistakes of others is better.

Growth is all part of learning. I started to train at a very young age, so my habits and conditioning have been forged over a long period of time. But in that time I've taken my fair share of wrong turns.

I used to think that taking whey protein would make me look like an IFBB* pro. To 15-year-old me, magazines were the holy grail of fitness material. Gurus of the past would say things that today have been thoroughly debunked.

More often than not, there are several ways of doing something and each of them may have their pros and cons – it's about finding out what's right for you.

So, mistakes are good, as long as you learn from them. And, the earlier you make mistakes, the faster you begin the process of elimination.

---

* International Federation of Bodybuilding and Fitness

USE THE POWER OF THE MIND

By unpicking errors, we can see where problems occurred. This is how successful businesses are created. This is how technology improves and it's also fundamental in scientific research and medicine. Somebody capitalizes on an idea that failed, or they identify what went wrong, and then they rectify it. Room for improvement is identified and so begins the evolution of something new.

There's no reason we can't do this personally, too. Look into your past, analyse bad habits and see where things can be improved. Identify what went wrong the last time you tried to lose weight, or why you never built muscle, or what you might be able to do next to improve your physique. You may fail or flail, but never give up.

So, is there a way to avoid making those mistakes to begin with?

The simple answer is no. Errors are merely obstacles that should make us change direction or try something new. The key is to change tack if something doesn't work, rather than give up altogether. So for example: you've set your goal to workout every morning at 7am before the day starts, but you keep missing it, or are feeling exhausted. Why not change the time, and see if that works better with your rhythm? We're not "giving up", we're adapting to still reach the same goal.

The goals I've mentioned above: getting fit or losing weight and keeping it off, require long-term action. They are journeys not destinations. I know that sounds clichéd, and it is. If you work hard to get fit and then just give up, those results will quickly fade. Chances are, once you start to see results, you'll want more, but your body will work against you. This is where the goalposts need to be moved, the training increased. This is time for re-evaluation. This is where people can rebound and fall off, or at the other end of the scale, look to synthetics to keep the results coming.

DO A SELF-APPRAISAL

I guarantee you this: every person you see parading their physique on stage or online has developed their own training protocols by testing, tinkering and also borrowing from others. If something doesn't work, try something else. Just don't give up.

And don't throw yourself under the bus because you ate something bad, or because you went off the rails for a bit. Beating yourself up will only make it worse. Instead of focusing on what you've done wrong, put that energy into working harder. Use those extra calories as fuel. Work a little harder to put it right.

Combat stress with mindfulness

Stress is a killer. Chances are, it may already be ingrained in your DNA. It is certainly part of mine. The human mind is not conditioned to receive the vast amount of information we receive nowadays and this causes congestion. We are often not fully aware of how much this affects us emotionally.

Having an aesthetic physique, or striving for one, can place enormous stress on both the body and the mind – especially if you're already predisposed to getting stressed – and I wholeheartedly encourage you to take action to address this. We can all reduce stress by adapting or introducing certain lifestyle practices.

Practicing mindfulness, for instance, is a tried-and-tested method that can help to lower cortisol levels in the body and allow you to get some inner peace. Mindfulness has also been shown to release tension, improve mental resilience, lower blood pressure, improve digestion, aid the autonomic nervous system and control pain.

So, what is mindfulness?

Simply put, mindfulness is paying full attention to something and slowing down to really notice what you are doing at any given time. That's why it's often referred to as being fully present and "in the moment". If any thoughts or sensations arise to distract you while you are doing so, the aim is to observe these thoughts objectively with an attitude that is non-judgemental, curious and kind.

You can practise all kinds of daily tasks mindfully to help get your stress under control. Start by taking 10 minutes in the morning, or at any time in the day, to sit quietly and just focus on your breathing, noticing each breath. It helps to clear your mind of clutter. You can also walk mindfully, eat mindfully and even sit mindfully and, over time, your mind will become less busy and you'll find it easier to focus on your tasks and goals.

As well as using tools like mindfulness, regular exercise itself is a great stress-buster, as is treating your body with respect in general. Getting quality sleep and eating clean, nutrient-dense food will give you a strong foundation from which to build your body and boost its performance and strength.

The choices I have made in life mean I have adopted a healthier way of living, and this helps me to keep stress at bay. Understand that, if a person is an alcoholic and they stop drinking, it doesn't mean they are cured. They are just in control of that situation. If stress is genetic, or if it runs in your family, then don't be afraid to tackle it. Be prepared. If stress comes at you unexpectedly, as it so often does, ensure you have measures in place to help manage your life effectively.

For many people that might be the gym. Usually, this is the one place people with stressful jobs and lives can go to get away from everything, to unwind. Just make sure your workouts don't increase your stress levels. And if you are in any doubt about being able to control your stress, always seek medical advice.

DO A SELF-APPRAISAL

SOCIAL MEDIA DETOX / CHALLENGE

SOCIAL MEDIA CAN BE GREAT, BUT IT CAN ALSO BE TOXIC AT TIMES AND CAN CAUSE HUGE AMOUNTS OF STRESS.

How many hours each week do you spend on your laptop, mobile phone or tablet, or all three?

How often do you open up an app and suddenly find yourself getting annoyed or outraged by a news story, or by something a total stranger has said online.

Do a little assessment – and be honest with yourself – about how much of your social media time is a positive experience for you and how much is just the opposite.

If your connections with the online world are more negative than positive, try reducing your screen time a little. In fact, most of us probably spend too long online, so try reducing it anyway.

Delete certain apps so you are not inclined to check your phone before bed, or as soon as you wake up in the morning.

Try turning your phone off for an hour each evening and having a mini detox, or spend one evening a week without it altogether.

Or set yourself a challenge instead. Every time you're tempted to pick up your phone, do ten push ups instead. You'll soon feel the temptation begin to fade.

Find the path to success

Success looks different to everyone, which makes it somewhat difficult to measure.

Success is a fluid concept. It doesn't matter if you consider yourself successful right now. What really matters is whether your daily choices are putting you on the path to continued success.

While some people rest on their perceived notion of success, others like to stress and complain about their current situation, but when pressed are not doing anything to better their lives.

The way I look at it, success equals progress. And progress can be measured.

Success is the product of building and continuing positive daily habits, not once-in-a-lifetime transformations. So, whatever success looks like to you, continue to seek it out. Strive for that feeling of progress and accomplishment.

Anything can be considered a success, even if it feels like only the smallest of victories. A win is a win.

In this part of the book we have explored the power of your mind and the many benefits you will see if you harness its power and bring it on board as you look to improve your body and your wellbeing.

In Part 3, we will examine how you can put these skills into practice, to create a plan that will help you achieve total mind and body fitness.

DO A SELF-APPRAISAL

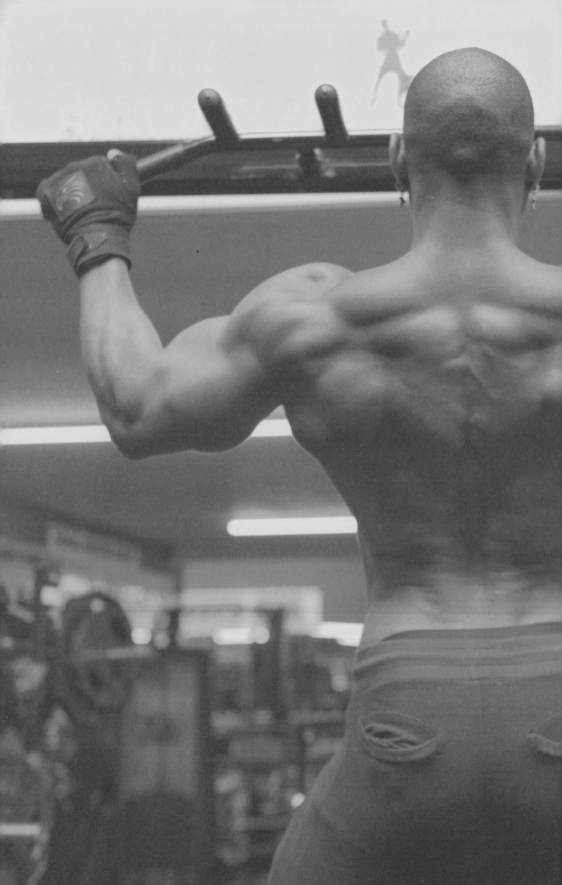

PART
3

A Plan for Self-Improvement

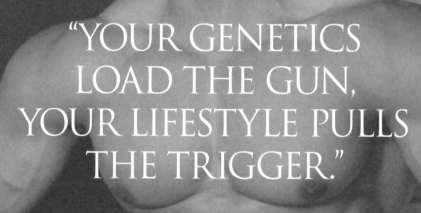

"YOUR GENETICS
LOAD THE GUN,
YOUR LIFESTYLE PULLS
THE TRIGGER."

Mehmet Oz

CHAPTER 5

UNDERSTAND YOUR POTENTIAL

While success can be measured by charting progress, the idea of human potential suggests the measurement of one's absolute peak. But what is this, exactly?

The route to peak performance and conditionioning can seem endless. Show me a human being who appears to be at the top of their game, and I'll bet they still see room for improvement.

Human potential is largely down to perceived boundaries. If you fill your mind with limitations, you will find little room for growth. Like success, we all have different ideas of peak potential. One person's idea of a big house will be another person's idea of solitary confinement. If a man has the desire to be a free diver, he may be limited by his ability to hold his breath for long periods of time.

So, what I'm saying here is, don't compare yourself to others. Only compare yourself to who you were last night, last week or last year. You may never know how far you can really push yourself, but often it's the desire to push yourself toward this unobtainable goal that will fuel your drive. Don't aim for one goal and stop when you get there – your potential is limitless. Just keep moving forward.

Genetics

I have spent over 25 years of my life fitting pieces of the puzzle together to try to understand what makes my body tick and, most importantly, what makes it perform at its best.

I am fascinated by the continual scientific advances that enable us to optimize our individual potential. One area that particularly interests me is genetics – the study of our inherited characteristics – and DNA testing. We all have DNA, but what makes us unique is how it's all combined together. Likewise, we all know that keeping physically active benefits us. But do we know what type of activity or diet we should be taking to best suit our individual body's needs?

Back when I decided to hang up the tiny trunks, I began working as a personal trainer in a prestigious gym. One day, we were introduced to a company who could check our DNA, in order to identify personal genetic traits. Their test would explain what type of exercises would be most suitable for us as individuals, and what types of foods we should consume or avoid. This would help optimize our training. It was the beginning of something that's been vital to my fitness journey. If you don't know where you've come from, how do you know how far you can go?

There are several reputable companies who offer a simple DNA test to provide a genetic profile and report that covers all the important markers to help us make the best diet and fitness decisions. Some examples would be carbohydrate sensitivity, antioxidant needs, coeliac predisposition (important if you're a big fan of grains), saturated fat sensitivity and caffeine sensitivity. In addition, they can look at your power to endurance ratio and recovery profile, and offer diet recommendations tailored to your specific needs. These things all add up. They all make a difference. You can also find out about the genetic chronotype that informs your circadian rhythm helping you to balance your activities and sleep accordingly.

I personally feel this is truly remarkable stuff and it has helped me make some vital choices for my lifestyle.

CORE PRINCIPLE 5

GET TO KNOW YOURSELF, INSIDE AND OUT

Like a machine, the body has a very specific set of design functions. It has been created with purpose, and that is to survive at all cost. In order to get the best from your body you must listen to it and respect it. And the first step is to learn as much about it as you can.

It takes time and patience to reach one's peak. We try and we fail. We try again and then we adapt. We try again and then we improve. This is how we evolve, through trial and error.

This is also how muscle is built. By breaking it down, allowing it to repair. Thus, it becomes stronger. It is a complex process that begins with some simple knowledge. Not just an understanding of the nuts and bolts of nutrition and exercise, but through knowledge of YOUR limitations. Knowing WHAT WORKS and WHAT DOESN'T.

›› Log the food you eat and make an honest assessment.

›› Take a DNA test or a micro-biome test, if you can afford it and want to look into the types of food you might be intolerant to, or the vitamins you might be lacking.

How important are genetics in bodybuilding?

Our genes play an important role in predicting possibility, but they do not fully define outcome. For example, if your body's response to the "a-actinin-3" protein in your muscle fibres is dominant, then you may be able to put on muscle quicker. Similarly, the ACE gene (Angiotensin Converting Enzyme) is responsible for blood flow. Having it could put you at an advantage, as it means more oxygen reaches the tissues and more nutrients will be carried to the muscles.

UNDERSTAND YOUR POTENTIAL

EPIGENETICS

Epigenetics is the study of the combination of your genes and how they are expressed. It's all about how the information in your genes is actually used by your body's cells, and how this is influenced by environment. Our genes can be considered the hardware or blueprint of our bodies, and our epigenetics are affected by lifestyle and choices, making them the software. The software instructions can change over time through healthy living or pursuing an unhealthy lifestyle.

This emerging and exciting field of science shows that, again, your genes are not the end of the story – so much of it is up to you.

Epigenetics looks at what happens to your body over the course of your life. Certain genes may be advantageous for you, but genetic mutations can also occur due to bad diet, environment, stress, and lack of sleep, etc. These can be detrimental over time. So, while genetics do give certain people advantages, they are neither a pre-written destiny, nor a substitute for hard work.

Genetics and me

I've proved to myself that with discipline and extreme focus, good things are obtainable. I like the saying, "The harder you work the luckier you get" because I do get people that say I'm "lucky" because of my genes. They work just as hard, but the results are not the same.

So, maybe I am lucky. Maybe I'm genetically more gifted than some. But, it wasn't genetics that made me place instant gratification to one side while others celebrated small achievements. Genetics didn't make me stop drinking on my birthday. Or make me continue intermittent fasting while I was at an all-inclusive resort on holiday. Genetics didn't make me use a tall travel backpack to carry my shopping and cycle uphill instead of using my car.

And genetics certainly didn't make me invest a large sum of money on educating myself in self-development on different levels of fitness.

Determine your body type

Our genes play a fundamental role in defining our base fitness and size and this is especially apparent where body shape is concerned. Losing weight, gaining muscle, building strength – these things can feel like an uphill battle for some people and not so hard for others, and this will largely be down to body type.

The three main textbook definitions of body type are mesomorph, ectomorph and endomorph and they are defined as follows:

›› **A mesomorph is muscular and well built with a high metabolism**

›› **An ectomorph is lean and has difficulty building muscle**

›› **An endomorph is bigger with a higher percentage body fat and higher tendency to store it.**

Most people will fall in between two categories, or may have many traits from one body type, with perhaps a little bit from another.

Depending on your main physical goal or the sport you may be interested in, I think all three body types have advantages and disadvantages.

If your goal is singularly to build lean muscle mass then, of course, being a mesomorph is the ideal base.

A MESOMORPH has the ability to grow muscle and keep body fat off, which is the desired effect for most bodybuilders. Mesomorphs' testosterone levels are often high, as is their growth hormone level. This combination is fundamental in the building of lean muscle.

AN ECTOMORPH has a slimmer body shape, which is ideal for long distance running. Their frames are lighter, so any impact when the feet hit the ground will be minimal. Ectomorphs tend to have a higher sympathetic nervous system, so their bodies burn calories at a higher fuel rate. This means it has less chance of gaining fat and muscle, compared to a mesomorph.

ENDOMORPHS have the largest body type and have a strong predisposition for gaining both muscle and fat. Endomorphs are usually thick-set or stocky. Their physiques are ideal for sports where strength and power are pre-requisites such as bodybuilding, wrestling, rugby and power lifting.

Don't be defined by your age

Your age does not define you, but it does have an impact on who you are and what you are capable of achieving.

Why not be super healthy and look great at the same time? Remember, I am in my 40s. I've never felt or looked better since I've been alive. Age is just a number *if* taking care of yourself is your number one priority.

A PLAN FOR SELF-IMPROVEMENT

Your biological age – the age of your body, your organs, your physical power – tells you whether your clock is ticking at a normal speed, or faster, or if you have successfully hacked the biological code and slowed down your degeneration through healthy habits.

It is completely possible for your biological age to be younger than your actual age. This again is all down to good health and sensible life choices. There are plenty of places where you can check your biological age online.

Atrophy and Hypertrophy

Atrophy is a state of degeneration, where the body's functionality declines though age or overuse. Sometimes organs fail, as does cognitive function which is known as Pathological Atrophy.

Where muscular development is concerned, Atrophy is the wasting away of muscle tissue through hormonal imbalance.

This can be caused simply by age, but also by injury, illness, poor health or sedentary lifestyle.

The opposite is called Hypertrophy. Hyper, meaning "above beyond" and trophy, from the Greek word trephein, which means to nourish.

This is essentially growth, or an increase in muscle cells which ultimately means size. Building muscle.

With age comes fear. Fear of the unknown. Fear of starting something new. But remember, fear also protects us from danger. Under threat, our brains resort to survival instincts and these instincts become more sensitive with age. This is why it's so hard to break bad habits, or instil new routines, especially as we get old.

The human brain is primitive, but our actions don't have to be. We all endure pitfalls while we search for fulfilment and success. Some people will forgo their goals due to injury, where some will encounter pain and work through it. Aging can cause both physical and mental limitations, while society has also conditioned us to believe we are in our "prime" when we are young, and that decline is the inevitable outcome of growing old. But by altering the chemistry of our bodies through biohacking, we can increase testosterone levels and begin to turn back the clock. Or at least slow it down.

TESTOSTERONE

Testosterone is a natural steroid and male sex hormone that is key in producing muscle mass and bone density due to protein synthesis. It helps with muscle maintenance. The more you have the more muscle you can keep.

Your testosterone levels (also knows as T-levels) naturally begin to decline as you age and this can begin from the age of 30. The older you get, the more your testosterone lowers and with it your strength and muscle mass. It can also lead to bone frailty, too.

Low testosterone levels can also affect mood, your ability to keep strong erections, as well as sexual appetite and libido.

A healthy diet with nutrient dense foods (such as eggs and quality beef) can improve testosterone levels, as can good sleep, low stress and resistance training. Compound lifts and training the legs can also improve T-levels. The stronger you are, the more chance you have of raising your levels. Essentially, lifestyle and diet will determine whether you keep a healthy testosterone level or not.

If you are concerned at all about your testosterone levels, please see a doctor for further advice.

CHAPTER 6

HOW CHEMISTRY INFORMS BIOLOGY

When we talk about the body, what we're really talking about is biology. Likewise, when we talk of diet, we are really concerned with the body's chemistry – the effect food has on us.

Our biology is essentially the hardware while its chemistry is the software. The diet you follow has all the binary codes, the data to operate the hardware. As long as you use food that is compatible with the hardware (your body), then you will become a far more resourceful, more formidable machine.

In this chapter, we'll look at some of the key biological processes related to health and fitness – your blood sugar, body fat and eating regimes – to better understand how you can support your body to optimize its functionality.

Most people just think of food as fuel to feed hunger, or as a treat. But, selecting where macronutrients come from can determine how food is processed by the body, so let's look at food intake a little more carefully.

Control your blood sugar

The body's main source of energy is glucose. Glucose (or blood sugar) is stored in the liver and the muscles as a substance called glycogen which is obtained when carbohydrates are broken down and enter the bloodstream.

Different foods affect this process in different ways. For example, the body might feel tired after food – especially shortly after consuming foods loaded with sugar or food high in starch. What most people would call a "sugar crash".

To better illustrate this: 175 grams (6oz) of carbs from two different sources can alter your body chemistry in significantly different ways. Eating 175g (6oz) of french fries, for instance, will flood your blood stream with glucose. This will most likely spike your insulin (*see below*), due to the higher starch content of potato. Short term, this isn't something to be too concerned about, but long term may cause weight gain, damage to organs and perhaps even type 2 diabetes.

Asparagus meanwhile is filled with nutrients and less natural sugar. It contains folate which is good for cell development. It also contains vitamin K which is good for the immune system, vitamin C which aids the formation of collagen, and vitamin E which protects cell membranes. Asparagus is also fibrous, so it feeds your microbiome, as well. Asparagus will therefore produce less glucose.

What happens when insulin spikes

Insulin is a hormone released by the pancreas and it works to stabilize glucose levels in the blood.

Insulin forces the body to go through different phases. You may feel lethargic or your cognitive abilities may suffer after consuming large amounts of sugar or starch.

If your insulin is spiked too often, which is normally the case when the bloodstream is flooded with starchy / sugary foods on a regular basis, a person can become insulin resistant which may cause both health and / or weight implications.

Become "crash" resistant

When the muscles and the liver become full and cannot hold any more glycogen, the next step is for the body to convert it to fat. This allows the body to take on more carbs as fuel. This is why a high-carb diet combined with little exercise, especially the muscle-building type, can lead to unhealthy weight gain and, potentially, diabetes.

However, the more *muscle* you have the more glycogen you can potentially burn per day. And when the muscles become depleted, the liver can free up some more glycogen which then provides the body with extra energy.

This is why creating a muscular core and lifting heavy weights will aid fat loss. Your body will effectively become more efficient at processing calories as energy. This means you can indulge in sugary foods selectively and not suffer the consequences (*see* pages 114–5).

Getting to know more about your blood sugar and insulin levels, and why they are so important in terms of fat storage, is essential if you are determined to change your body composition. Knowing which foods can spike insulin and have the potential to upset your body's chemistry will help you to target good and bad choices and enable you to focus on optimal health and also preventative health care.

A regular pattern of high blood sugar will have a detrimental effect on your health and can cause illness. Many diseases breed and thrive on carbohydrates, when they are consumed over-indulgently. Just knowing how your body responds can help you make informed decisions about food and hold you accountable.

 If in doubt, I would encourage you to get your blood sugar levels regularly tested – there are various inexpensive testing kits on the market or you can consult your doctor.

CORE PRINCIPLE 6

INCREASE YOUR METABOLIC FLEXIBILITY (MF)

Metabolic flexibility is the ability to respond or adapt to conditional changes in metabolic demand.

Metabolic flexibility aids the dispersion of glucose within the body. This stops the body storing it as fat.

There are four metrics that help us control our glucose. These are:

1. Activity level
2. Muscle mass
3. Physical fitness
4. Physically active

The benefits of having greater muscle mass means you will have a smaller insulin spike than those with less muscle density. The more muscle mass you have, the better you will be at disposing of glucose.

If you are physically active before eating, or partake in one rigorous workout, your insulin sensitivity will increase (for up to 48hrs), in essence diluting any spike in your blood sugar levels.

Fasting will also aid Metabolic Flexibility, as does carbohydrate timing – eating a larger quantity of your daily carbohydrate allowance around a big workout will allow the body to process the glycogen produced.

Understand body fat 🎙

Our bodies are affected by the food sources we consume and the stress we put upon our muscles and our bones. The food we eat creates energy (as calories) and, as I've just explained, this is stored as glycogen until our body can hold no more and it is turned to fat. So, unless we are in a caloric deficit, or we sufficiently burn more calories than we consume, we will increase our body fat.

As we get older, our fat cells expand and take on fat more easily – and so it becomes much harder to lose weight (fat) with age. If you think of each of your fat cells as a balloon. When new, a balloon has to be stretched and takes a great deal of effort to fill it with air and force it to expand. But over time, and if repeatedly expanded, the balloon begins to lose its shape. Its outer structure weakens and it becomes a lot easier to fill with air and will expand more, as well.

This is how fat cells work. When we are young, gaining weight can be difficult. This is particularly prevalent in a lot of young men who may eat excessively in a bid to gain weight, and then increase their calorie intake when they start to train. But as these young men get older, their bodies will begin to change. The fat cells expand and become harder to clear. When fat is lost, the cells instead fill with water. This is why men and women of a certain age can hold on to stubborn fat or get that bloated appearance.

Subcutaneous and visceral fat

There are two different kinds of fat deposits that the body stores in different ways: subcutaneous fat and visceral fat.

Subcutaneous fat is the visible type of fat that sits between the muscle tissue and the skin. For some people it can cause a lot of worry, mainly because it is visible. One problem with subcutaneous fatty tissue is that it tends to store a lot of toxins, too. When people lose body fat they tend to get sick shortly after or their immune system can become compromised. This is because the toxins are released into the blood stream. The level of toxicity in the fat will determine how serious it can be for the person.

Visceral fat tends to surround the organs and it is not as visible as subcutaneous fat. This doesn't mean it's not there and that it shouldn't be a concern. Chances are, if your waist is big and it's not through gymnastics and intense core exercises then I would say this is serious and you should clean up your lifestyle.

A big stomach or gut is a sign of visceral fat. Any fat surrounding your vital organs will have a profound effect on your health and can leave you at high risk of heart disease and Type 2 diabetes.

However, you can also be visually skinny and still hold a high level of visceral fat. A man with an ectomorph body type (eats like a dinosaur but looks like an envelope sideways) can be light in weight but fat in the gut, which will still put his health at risk.

Although I would never say it's important to have a six-pack, I would say that you have less chance of holding toxins and inflammations if you don't carry fat in your mid-section. Your body's metabolic flexibility (*see* page 84) will be much better the leaner you are.

Calorie expenditure and fat loss

Learning a little about fat and how it is stored in the body helps us to understand how losing weight and losing fat are not necessarily the same thing. Typically, when calorie intake surpasses energy usage, this will result in weight gain. If intake falls below your daily resting calorie allowance (BMR, *see* page 88), this will conversely result in fat loss.

BODY MASS INDEX

A broad indicator of whether or not you carry too much weight is to work out your Body Mass Index (BMI). This is a system that works on a ratio of height to weight, and if your weight is not in alignment with your height you will be considered overweight or even obese.

However, this BMI system is flawed, as a person can be heavy in weight and low in body fat because they have built a large amount of lean muscle tissue through resistance training. Still, it is important to know where you sit on the BMI, as many formulas for working out calorie intake will require it.

There are several online calculators where you can check your BMI, such as: www.nhs.uk/live-well/healthy-weight/bmi-calculator/

THERMOGENESIS

Losing weight on the scales will not necessarily happen if you are working out and building muscle. However, by increasing the amount of exercise you do, you will lose fat, which is generally a good thing. As we exercise, the body goes through a process known as thermogenesis. The word "thermogenic" means heat-producing. When your body burns calories, it generates more heat, which in turn boosts your metabolism and burns fat.

CATABOLISM

If you think food deprivation is the key to weight control and you purposely starve yourself, in effect not fuelling your body sufficiently, you can cause the body to break down muscle for fuel, instead. Losing muscle is an example of catabolism. Catabolism basically means the breaking down of a molecule – whether that is fat, protein or glucose. Your body doesn't like this and so it will fight back, in order to retain as much weight as possible, hitting the emergency switch to slow down your metabolism causing your body to hold on to more calories or weight. So, be aware that cutting calories from your diet too quickly is likely to have the adverse effect.

Create an eating regime

Your diet is merely how you chose to deliver nutrition to your body. But, selecting the right diet and meal plan is a lot like picking the perfect vacation spot. Much of it depends on external variables, such as the time of year, how hard or little you might be training, if you are a vegetarian or a vegan or have certain food intolerances – these are the kinds of things only you will know.

BASAL METABOLIC RATE (BMR)

To calculate your required calorie intake, you need to work out your Basal Metabolic Rate (BMR). This is the number of calories your body requires to sufficiently maintain function while at rest.

BMR is essentially your body's metabolism, so any increase to your metabolic weight, such as exercise, will increase your BMR. Understanding your BMR will allow you to determine your daily calorie needs, dependent on whether you want to gain or lose weight.

There are several online calculators, such as www.active.com/fitness/calculators/bmr, which can help you work out your BMR when you input your height, gender, age and weight. Once you have determined your BMR, you can then monitor how many calories a day you need to consume.

Understanding your body in relation to the diet you should follow is like unlocking a secret code. At least, that's what it might seem like to begin with. But in essence, it's only a matter of science.

To understand our need for food, I think there are no better teachers than our ancestors. Our human ancestors survived with large periods of fasting. Meat, dairy and grains were not readily available until farming was introduced. We were scavengers and opportunists before we were hunter-gatherers and eventually agriculturists.

Nowadays there is too much choice. We have become spoiled and greedy and we eat for pleasure more than out of necessity, and this has big implications for our overall health and fitness.

You will probably find yourself following a combination of diets, after trying and trialling several different eating plans. Some may be more successful than others, and you may find yourself flagging at times, but until you try certain things you won't know what works best for your lifestyle and body type.

If your overall goal is muscle growth, then you will probably be best served with a diet consisting of small regular meals that include a decent amount of protein combined with an appropriate amount of good carbs and fats.

If your goal is to get lean, then a low-carb or ketogenic diet will work best, possibly with an element of fasting thrown in. This is typically the combination of diets that I follow.

On the following pages I take a look at some of the common types of eating regimes associated with bodybuilding: calorie deficit, the ketogenic diet, fasting and time-restricted eating and any one, or a combination of these, should help you to lose body fat.

Calorie deficit

This is the simplest and most obvious of all dieting principles, yet, sometimes, it's the most difficult one to follow. Calories and energy work in harmony. The more calories you consume, the more energy you need to expend to prevent those calories being stored as fat in the body. If you remain in a calorific deficit and expend the appropriate amount of energy, you should lose weight.

This seems simple and, in theory, it is. However, it works best when you also consume as little processed foods as possible. This is because pre-packaged foods come with many hidden additives – sugars, trans fats, MSG – all of which, over time, will inhibit fat loss. So, you might think you are in a calorific deficit, when in fact you are in a surplus.

Put simply, the less factory interference, the better the food. Building muscle requires quality protein, but it also requires other nutrients, too. Many people focus heavily on the macro-nutrients and forget micro-nutrients, such as zinc, which is good for testosterone support and boosts the immune system. Magnesium, as well, which is one of the most abundant minerals in the body, is great for improving sleep.

We need to understand that diet is more than just calories. All foods contain messages that are interpreted in different ways by the body.

CULTIVATE GOOD HABITS

Like bad habits, most bad diets stem from your childhood. My dad was poor, so my diet was too. Before going to work, my dad would eat bread and butter, so this habit was handed down. My idea of healthy eating back then was adding some processed chicken and a bit of salad to a sandwich. But, over time I learned about the benefits of good nutrition. Watching videos of the first competition I took place in, I realize I had no idea about nutrition back then – my diet was atrocious. I used to eat half a loaf of bread, or readymade soup and corned beef straight from the tin.

The human body is a complex machine that adapts quickly to new stimuli, but it will also react just as quickly to bad nutrition. If you make a conscious effort to establish a good habit of working out three or four days a week, you will soon reap rewards – especially if you didn't work out at all to begin with. Likewise, if you start (or don't kick) a bad habit, it can become detrimental over time. Eating that "protein bar" packed with sugars, every day, will negate fat loss and derail progress.

If all of your carbohydrates come from chips, or all of your fats come via pizza, this will not only have a detrimental effect to your long-term goals, but it will also affect your cravings for unhealthy food. Starchy, fatty foods are okay in moderation, but because they have very little nutritional content, if incorporated into your everyday eating plan they will eventually derail your efforts in the gym as well.

The ketogenic diet

The ketogenic diet, or keto, is the process whereby you are essentially tricking your body into burning fat for energy instead of glucose (*see* page 82). This is because a keto diet consists of high fat, moderate protein and a very low intake of carbohydrates (and, of course, refined sugar). The idea is that by feeding your body only fat, it will adapt to utilize this as its primary energy source, and will then tap into its own fat reserves as well.

This can happen only if you reduce the amount of carbohydrates you eat so that your body will search for an additional fuel source. The general keto rule is to consume fewer than 50 grams of carbohydrates a day (or 20g if we are talking about a very strict keto diet). Your body will then not be able to rely on carbs to get its energy. Instead, it depends on ketones, and this is a process known as ketosis.

If there is no indication of sugar in the bloodstream the pancreas will not produce insulin. Instead, the liver takes your fatty acids and produces chemicals called ketones in your bloodstream so that you have the energy to live.

Your body stores fat, so your liver is happy to process this as an alternative fuel. In fact, it is a very clean form of energy because the brain is able to utilize ketones effectively, and once your body becomes fat-adapted your mind becomes much clearer. Again this is down to the ketones.

However, in order to follow a ketogenic diet efficiently you must fully commit to it. It can take up to ten days for your body to switch into fat-burning mode (this is where you become fat-adapted). You must be incredibly strict with what you eat as even a small amount of carbohydrates can send you out of ketosis.

Generally, people cycle periods of ketosis with re-feeds – these are essentially days or weekends when you eat a regular diet and replenish some glycogen.

Thankfully, once you have become fully fat-adapted, your body will remember this state and it will be much easier to switch back into fat burning mode during your next period of ketosis.

Fasting

Fasting is simply a set period of not eating, and maybe not drinking as well. It can be for a few hours or longer. Many people try fasting because they want to lose weight, predominantly fat. That in itself is probably a potent enough reason to look into it.

Eating over too many hours of the day creates oxidative stress within the body, which can lead to premature aging. Oxidative stress is an imbalance between free radicals in the body, which cause cell damage, and the antioxidants that combat this.

Long resting periods from eating allow the body time to repair and regain balance in this area. Fasting also aids in the improvement of insulin sensitivity and can help resolve low-grade inflammation.

Fasting also allows your body to produce more ketones (*see* pages 91-2), which use your own body fat as energy instead of glycogen.

INTERMITTENT FASTING (IF)

Intermittent fasting is the process of going for a set number of hours each 24-hour day without food. This might be 14, 16 or 18 hours, for example. And in the remaining time (your eating window, *see* below), you might consume one or two meals. You can also restrict your eating window thereby curbing the amount of food you consume over a 24-hour period (restricting calories and forcing your body to tap into fat reserves for fuel).

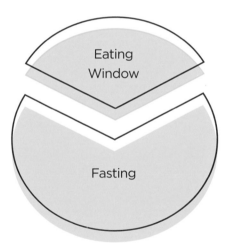

Basic 8/16 eating window

My own intermittent fasting journey has been amazing. My discipline has improved. My appreciation of the taste of food has increased. And giving myself just a small window to eat in has allowed me more time to do other things.

It wasn't all plain sailing. As soon as begin to restrict meal times, or calories in general, you suddenly want to consume ALL CALORIES at once. The mental struggle is real. Especially if you've been conditioned to eat within 30 minutes of waking followed by another meal (lunch) just a few hours later.

I used to eat 5–6 meals a day with regular snacks over a span of 14–15 hours. Now, I regularly consume one or two meals over a 4- or 6-hour period, and the meals I eat are much more nutrient-dense than those I would consume if eating at regular intervals. I don't feel my strength has been compromised. If anything, my endurance has improved.

Since intermittent fasting, my body shape has tightened up, and my mental clarity has also improved. I do sometimes miss that slightly fuller look you get with eating six meals a day, but I believe the benefits of fasting are far greater.

Fasting allows me to focus on my digestive system for longevity, essentially giving it time to recuperate, which then allows my body to recover more effectively from exercise.

Fasting isn't a new fad either. Our ancestors conformed to lengthy fasting periods, eating for short periods before rest. The sun would set and melatonin would kick in. During this time, their metabolisms would slow down and the digestive system and insulin would prepare for rest and recovery. While in this fasting period, self-cleansing in the body and brain detoxification would take place. They would need to be alert by the morning, in case they would need to flee from a wild animal or an enemy, so waking up and feeling sluggish wasn't an option.

Restricting your eating time (not necessary calories) gives your body the rest and recovery time it needs to make you a stronger, energy efficient and more productive person. Reducing your eating window to at least 12 hours to start off with will potentially extend your life and will also give you more time to do other things right now. Remember: this is all about a lifestyle not a diet!

Besides increasing your energy levels, eating less often can naturally stimulate HGH (human growth hormone). This is the hormone that, like testosterone, can aid muscle growth and help with fat loss. If you are HGH deficient as an adult you may experience higher levels of body fat, loss of muscle tissue and decreased bone mass. Eating the right foods at the right time, along with exercise and weight training, will help naturally stimulate HGH and testosterone.

HOW TO STRUCTURE YOUR EATING WINDOW
In theory, the ideal balance of exercise with a good diet to offset your lifestyle, should look something like this:

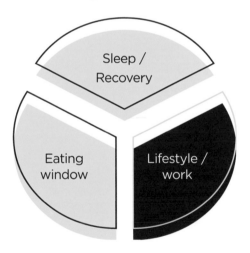

8/16 eating window

With 8 hours for sleep, your eating window comprises of half the remaining 16 hours (making it a little easier to adhere to).
For most people, I think it's easier to split the day into four. The average person might spend around six hours at work, with perhaps six hours of quality sleep (not ideal, but how many people really get eight hours of uninterrupted sleep a night?). Everything else is taken

up with leisure or life admin. If you have children or care for somebody else, then this window may be even shorter. With that said, your day will probably look more like this:

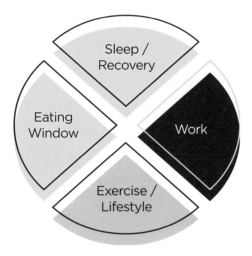

6/18 eating window

EATING WINDOW: This should comprise of a balance of nutrition, fuel or food which is as important as exercise.

EXERCISE: Anything that consists of movement and energy consumption. From a gentle walk to rigorous exercise.

REST: This is an important part of exercise. But I mean "recovery" and not just lounging around on the sofa eating junk.

LIFESTYLE: When I say "lifestyle", I refer to everything else, from work, to socializing and entertainment. This is usually where we slip up, hence why this portion of the day is probably the hardest to adhere to a fast.

Work may lead to stress. For example, long hours of being sedentary – sitting at a desk – may also contribute to a poor diet. Likewise, our home and social lives tend to be times where we are free and often careless with diet choices. We may also be sedentary (sitting at home, watching the television with the family while they are eating snacks, so we are more likely to indulge, as well).

Unless you're planning on competing or want to make it your life's work, as I have, then what you really want is balance and moderation. If you have the time, that's great (because you'll probably need it).

In practice, the balance of my day looks more like this (note how small my eating window is:

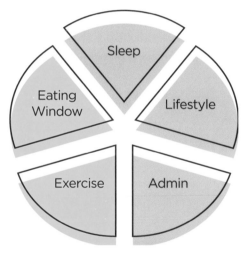

1/5 eating window

For most of us, the shape of our day will be entirely different, and that's okay. So long as you have time to incorporate exercise and diet into your life, then that's a start.

Looking after you health should factor into your day, regardless. Without it your quality of life will definitely suffer, so don't make excuses and find the time to fit it in.

HOW CHEMISTRY INFORMS BIOLOGY

TIME RESTRICTED EATING (TRE)

TRE is essentially another incarnation of Intermittent Fasting which gives you a set time during a 24 hour period where you can consume your required daily calorie allowance.

Time Restricted Eating is a little less restrictive as it allows one to use amino acids, black coffee, herbs or MCT outside of the eating window, to accompany one's fast.

While I am in a fasting period, I might also take apoptogenic herbs to aid with my fast. These can help to mimic the benefits of the fast.

Over time I have condensed my eating pattern from a 16+ hour eating window down to just 4 hours. TRE allows me to focus on my digestive system for longevity, essentially giving it time to recuperate, which then allows my body recover more effectively.

To many this would seem utterly insane, but to me it makes perfect sense for my lifestyle.

For me, restricting my eating window (but not necessarily my calorie intake) gives my body the rest and recovery time it needs to make it stronger, and more energy efficient.

Try reducing your eating window to at least 12 hours to begin with and then slowly decreasing it. This will potentially increase your energy (once you adapt) and it will certainly feel as though you have more time to do other things as well.

CHAPTER 7

EATING TO PROMOTE MUSCLE GROWTH

In this chapter, we're going to talk about diet and nutrition. Eating well is a huge part of building your body, and the informed choices you make will give you the energy and resilience to take your fitness journey to the next level. We'll take a look at how to view your macros as well as the emerging field of good gut health. I'll also share some of my top diet hacks to help you navigate everyday temptations and show you how to eat smart to optimize your nutritional intake.

Eating to promote muscle growth requires a diet rich in high-quality protein but, like most things in life, it isn't as simple as just that. It calls for a holistic approach. As well as requiring a whole range of nutrients, your body needs to be in good shape to absorb them to maximum efficiency. For example, for effective absorption of protein, it's best to lose any excess body fat first, if you are holding it. Your body will then be more insulin-sensitive and metabolically flexible too. The leaner you are, the easier it will be to gain lean muscle, compared to someone who is holding lots of fat. But let's start by getting back to basics.

Track your macros

As we've already said, foods aren't made up of just one macro-nutrient, but are usually a combination of fats, carbohydrates or proteins. The best sources of nutrition for bodybuilding are always foods made from simple non-processed ingredients – the basic rule of thumb here is the less factory interference there is, the better the food. The amount of nutrients your body needs will also vary depending on muscle mass, age, gender, and body fat percentage, too.

Some people are constantly tracking their macros, checking exactly how many grams of protein, fat and carbs they consume in each meal every day. I think this can lead to obsessive tendencies around fitness and that actually, it's far more important to just focus on eating well. Deep down, we all know if we've eaten too much food, or if what we've eaten is going to be detrimental to our health, so I think for the most part people need to just focus on eliminating garbage food from their diets before considering how much of their daily intake comes from a set amount of protein, carbs and fats.

Many fitness professionals supplement their diets with whey protein from a tub and other unnatural substances, When I talk about 'clean food' I mean fresh, or whole foods. Meat without additives or flavourings that I prepare from ingredients that didn't come store-prepared. Eggs, rice, potatoes and fresh vegetables.

If you begin by cleaning up your diet and focusing on healthier eating to ensure your body works optimally, once you are used to eating the right kinds of food then you can progress to a stricter eating plan which may include tracking your macros. When you are ready for this step, there are many apps that will help you to log your food and exercise, and track your macros: for example, MyFitnessPal or MyPlate. Over time, the food and exercise choices you make will become instinctive and your body will become a fat-burning machine if you follow your daily routine.

Now let's look at macros in a little more detail.

Protein

Protein is the go-to food source for every fitness fanatic, gym enthusiast, athlete and bodybuildier. It is the essential macronutrient for building muscle and aiding recovery due to its abundance of amino acids – the basic constituents of protein.

People think more protein equals more gains, but this is not entirely true. Most protein is only 18–48 percent absorbed. So, rounding that up, 50 percent to 80 percent of all protein eaten is wasted. Considering the premium cost of protein sources, that's a diminishing return the more you consume!

The point I'm making here is one of efficiency. We want our blood to fill with amino acids and fuel the muscles. There are different theories to how many grams of protein you should consume. I recommend 1–1.5 grams (around 0.05oz) per kg of lean body mass, or up to 2.0g (0.07oz) per kg of body weight for bodybuilders or athletes involved in intense training. Sometimes though, it's a case of going by how you feel. If you feel satiated then take it as a sign to stop.

Consuming too much protein can have a detrimental effect (while fasting or on a very low carb diet) and can result in glycogenesis. This is where the protein we eat turns into sugar. As we've seen on pages 82-3, too much sugar will result in regular insulin spikes, and will then cause excess glycogen to be stored as fat if not used. This is of course self-defeating.

When consuming food, your body has to manufacture enzymes in order to break it down. The truth is, these enzymes can come from protein, and also from muscle. So, by overdoing your protein intake, you could end up compromising your own muscle mass. This is a worst-case scenario, but is something to consider for people who are much older, who have fewer digestive enzymes or lower muscle mass.

Another issue we have today is that much of the food we buy is deficient in natural enzymes. Either we kill most of them when we cook the food, or they have been damaged during the factory process. That again means we pay for this at our muscles' expense. We'll talk more about eating clean shortly but, for now, take this as another reason to ditch the ready meals.

EATING TO PROMOTE MUSCLE GROWTH

ENZYMES

There are three types of enzymes that the body requires, each used to digest the three types of macro.

›› Amylase is needed to digest carbohydrates.
›› Lipase is needed to digest fats.
›› Protease is needed to digest proteins.

Fats

Fats have had a bad rap for many years but, thankfully, people are now beginning to see the benefits of incorporating good fats into their diet. This is especially true when following a ketogenic diet and when you know how important it is to become fat-adapted (*see* page 91).

While trans fats and other processed fats such hydrogenated vegetable oil should be avoided, the introduction of good healthy fats should be a staple part of your diet. These include:

›› **Avocado**
›› **Eggs**
›› **Flax seed**
›› **Steak**
›› **Nuts**
›› **Peanut butter**
›› **Coconut oil**
›› **Olive oil**
›› **Butter (in moderation)**

It is worth remembering that while good for you, many natural fats are, in fact, high in calories, so you need to be mindful of portion size.

Carbohydrates

Not all carbs are equal. Some are a whole lot better for you than others.

You can't always reduce things to simple macros. Wholefood carbohydrates that contain fibre and nutrients – such as grains and fruits – are not that same as consuming the equivalent quantities of processed carbs, such as pasta, white bread or white rice.

As we've seen, certain foods elicit different biological responses and therefore will have different results.

Good carbs	Medium carbs	Starchy carbs (avoid)
Sweet potatoes	White potatoes	Pasta
Brown rice	White rice	White Bread
Green vegetables	Coloured veg / fruit	Pastry

Sugar

As we've seen (and all know), if consumed regularly in excess, sugar will convert to fat in the body. Even fructose – the sugar found in fruit – will cause your insulin to spike. Honey acts in the same way as a sugar, but it is a better alternative to refined sugar, especially in its raw state.

Glucose in a liquid form, such as soda or energy drinks high in sugar, or sweetened coffee, will be absorbed by the body much faster, creating a more prominent spike. Anything that spikes insulin too much and too often should really be avoided.

While it is difficult to avoid, and because many of us have become addicted to it, cutting out sugar altogether is going to be difficult. However, if you take it one step at a time and systematically eliminate refined sugar from your diet, I guarantee you will feel better for it and it will significantly improve your health.

ARTIFICIAL SWEETENERS

We all understand the dangers of consuming sugar, so we generally try to cut down, or we might switch to artificial sweeteners as an alternative. The way sweetener has been marketed makes it appetizing for those of us following healthy diets to reach our fitness goals, but we need to be aware of any potential dangers.

While they do not increase glucose, there is evidence to suggest that artificial sweetener may elicit an insulin spike, much like sugar, in order to metabolize what your body *thinks* is glucose. Essentially, it deceives your body, so is best avoided, or at least limited, if possible.

There are natural alternatives, such as stevia, which are derived from natural sugars or polyols (sugar alcohol).

THERE IS MORE TO FOOD THAN MACROS

Diets that focus solely on macros (If It Fits Your Macros, for example) may say you can eat anything that falls within a specific food group or category – up and to a certain amount of calories – but I think the thing to consider is whether or not an individual food supports your overall health. A greasy hamburger may equate to a proportion of your fats, proteins and carbohydrates for the day, but consuming hamburgers daily is certainly unhealthy and will not help you with cravings either .

Conjuring up a little willpower and making good food choices is the only thing that will empower your health.

CRAVINGS

Cravings, I believe, are a primal thing. They can be a sign of emotional eating: if you crave a specific food such as crisps (potato chips), or fries it's often to fill an emotional gap rather than a physical one.

The problem we face today is that a lot of food contains added ingredients that are unnecessary but are geared toward making us want more. These foods are usually saturated with synthetic enhanced flavourings and are also calorie-dense.

Food companies will sell you whatever they can in order to win your vote and make you a returning customer. For example, food rich in emulsifier creates a nice texture to increase the pleasure of your eating experience. You will eat more simply because your brain will tell you this is pleasurable to eat.

Many processed foods, snacks or candy bars are not only nutrient-deprived but also disrupt your limbic brain which is responsible for letting you know whether you need to eat or want to eat. And the frequency with which you eat junk foods makes you want them even more. These cravings can lead you on a downward spiral, if you let them.

Eating more "bad" food than "good" feeds the steering wheel of your cravings: the more you eat, the more you want. You lose metabolic flexibility (*see* page 84) so, when your blood sugar levels drop your body only knows to keep it filled with glycogen to avoid starvation.

The best way to prevent cravings and overeating are by eating more protein, fibrous vegetables and healthy fats, and by drinking plenty of water. Healthy eating regimes such as a ketogenic diet (*see* page 91-2) and intermittent fasting (*see* pages 93-4) will also kill hunger pangs and cravings.

Five diet hacks

These tips are particularly useful if you are counting calories either in order to build your body to its optimum size or to lose a little weight.

1. DON'T BUY DIET FOODS

Foods such as diet bars, ready to eat meals, meal replacement drinks, etc., are basically garbage. This also includes foods that claim to be "low fat" or "reduced sugar". Just ask yourself, why is the sugar reduced? And reduced from what? Was there more sugar in the recipe to begin with? And if something is low fat, what's the problem with fat? I want fat in my diet – it's important.

Also, many foods in the supermarkets nowadays claim to be "high in protein". This type of marketing tricks you into believing these are healthy alternatives to other foods. Adding peanuts to something, for example, does not make it "high in protein". It may add SOME protein, but nuts are also extremely high in calories. If in doubt, always carefully check the food labels.

2. DON'T HAVE "BAD" FOOD IN YOUR HOUSE ON PURPOSE

Only buy what you need. If you're going to have a cheat meal on a specific day, go out and buy any sweet treats on that day and that day only. Chances are, if you buy it beforehand and it's sitting in your cupboard, you will become tempted to eat it. Avoid this temptation by simply not buying it in the first place.

3. AVOID GIVING YOURSELF UNREALISTIC GOALS

Telling yourself you're going to lose 15kg (40lbs) in two weeks by spending several hours a day in the gym is just completely unrealistic. If you attempt it, you're going to end up injured, or you will burn yourself out. A slow and steady approach always wins in the end.

4. DON'T BURN THE CANDLE AT BOTH ENDS

When you are trying to achieve a goal, it's best if you give it 100% of your attention. And to get fit you need to commit. If you are trying to build your body but also still prioritizing going out and spending your valuable time on social events, you are setting yourself up for failure.

If you give in to peer pressure to go out, chances are you will give in to temptation and you will give up on your goals, as well. You don't have to sacrifice everything – there's no fun in that – but you will need to sacrifice a few things in order to overhaul your life. That's why it's an overhaul. You're trying to change, not stay the same. You can add some fun stuff into your schedule but just make sure you are prioritizing your gym or exercise time above this.

5. BE HONEST WITH YOURSELF

If you are counting the calories, then stick to your chosen measurements. Your mind can't trick your body where calories are concerned. Don't add an extra helping here and there, hoping to get away with it. Those extras will all add up to failure.

Low-fat crisps / potato chips or biscuits / cookies containing oats are not a suitable source of carbohydrate. These foods contain hidden sugars and trans fats, which are empty calories.

Improve your gut health

Now let's take a look at a topic that's hot in health and nutrition right now, and let me ask you, do you understand your gut?

I'm forever looking to expand my knowledge around scientifically proven methods that can help me to achieve a better self through optimizing my health. Gut health is a fascinating subject but, surprisingly it's one that many people don't care about. In fact, the only time people seem to question their gut health is if they are feeling unwell or have discomfort in the stomach area.

The body contains trillions of bacteria, some of which are there to help you live. It's our job to feed them. If you eat bad food, you feed the bad bacteria and then your good bacteria ends up losing the battle and are suddenly outnumbered. If this happens, you are in trouble.

Some bacteria are responsible for metabolic fitness, intestinal barrier health, digestion efficiency and much more. To analyze your gut health, you might want to consider getting it tested professionally with a company such as Viome, to see if you have any unwanted parasites causing problems or if your gut is doing well.

My own report gave recommendations based on the activity of microbes in my gut. These are foods I personally either need to avoid, minimize or can continue eating. I was also given my own personal superfood list as well. This included artichokes, which are a prebiotic (food source for the good bacteria in your gut) and also contain inulin, a complex sugar that is converted by the gut into butyrate, which is great for digestion and has anti-inflammatory effects.

If you care about your health, then you should care about your gut. To know exactly how healthy or not you are, I definitely recommend getting a gut test.

Alongside this, I also recommend following a detox. Detoxing allows me to rid my system of many partially hydrogenated fats, wheat sources and caffeine, revitalizing my digestive system and my gut.

Food intolerance and inflammation

It's a great benefit if your body tells you that something you're eating isn't right for you, but if you don't know you are intolerant to something or you don't avoid it, your body will eventually rebel.

If you know you'll be going out and potentially eating foods that upset your gut, or you're out drinking with friends or family, then put a contingency plan in place. Sounds nuts, I know, but unless you heal after the damage you cause, more hits from harsh foods can trigger reactions that are hard to rectify.

You can take certain medicines, but there are also natural remedies that can aid gut inflammation. For example, turmeric and ginger, which are easily taken or added to meals or drinks, are known for their anti-inflammatory properties, and also help to remove toxins from your body. Turmeric is also known to help your gut biome.

Hydrogen water helps to kill damaging free radicals in the body. It also gives your body an antioxidant boost that helps increase energy, decrease inflammation and protect against disease.

In terms of intolerance, avoidance is always better than a cure. If you think you might be sensitive to certain foodstuffs, try an elimination diet to identify them or get yourself tested. It can make a huge difference to weight, energy levels and overall vitality, all of which you want to be functioning optimally if you are serious about building your body.

CORE PRINCIPLE 7

STICK TO CLEAN WHOLE FOODS

I know this may seem a strange concept to promote when many fitness professionals supplement their diets with whey protein from a tub and other unnatural substances. But by "clean" I mean fresh produce, or whole, foods. Meat without additives or flavouring that you cook yourself and hasn't come store-prepared. Eggs, brown rice, sweet potatoes and vegetables that are fresh and organic.

Processed or pre-prepared food such as sandwiches, ready-meals, even protein bars should be avoided, if possible. You only have to look at their lists of ingredients to see the additives, preservatives and extra "hidden" sugars.

Checking the labels on the food you eat will have a big impact on what you allow into your body. I don't mean the "Low Fat" label on the front (which more often than not means it will also contain more sugar), or the more recent fad of labelling something "High in Protein", because it has some peanuts in it.

I mean checking the nutrition matrix on the back. If something weighs 250g (9oz) and has 50g (1.8oz) of sugar, that's 20 percent of the overall nutritional value of that entire food item. This is not good.

Protein bars and milkshakes found in the supermarket are the fitness industry's equivalent of fast food, so always read the label before you buy and beware.

If in doubt, always go for the natural option.

Choose natural

Nature doesn't take sides. Nature doesn't have any favourites either. It treats everyone alike. Whatever seed you plant in the ground, nature will grow it. Whatever thoughts you plant in your mind, nature will grow them, as well.

People like to claim online that I've taken steroids and that I'd never be able to build a physique like mine without synthetics. There will always be doubters.

"But are you natural, Roger?"

I get asked this question more times than I care to remember. To be honest, I understand. I used to get frustrated when people asked me this question, but now I just shrug it off.

I don't take anything synthetic. I am and always have been natural. Of course, I look at my photos and I compare them to others who I know use PEDs (performance-enhancing drugs) – and I can see why many people choose to not believe me. I'm okay with that now. I don't make decisions in my life for the approval of others. I make my own health choices. I work hard to see how far I can push my fitness level and I teach others who are willing to learn from the mistakes that I've made and the things I've done right.

I choose to be natural because it benefits me and gives me the best chance to live a long life. I don't have enough knowledge about PEDs to use them but I have no problems with others who do. What other people do is up to them.

People who find it hard to believe it's naturally possible to achieve my level of fitness are often not as genetically blessed as I have been. It's also likely they haven't spent the last twenty or so years trying to build their physique. I do make use of natural vitamin and mineral-based supplements from time to time as part of my biohacking regimen, which you can read about in the next chapter.

I'd encourage everyone to build their body the natural way. Not only is it possible to get a great physique this way, but you are also supporting your all-round health by following a natural, nutritional and holistic approach.

My first port of call is always research. Learn about the body, and more specifically, your own body. Chances are, if you're not growing or putting on muscle, this may be down to your body type, but more likely it's because your diet and training is not quite right for you.

Let's take a look at some other uncomplicated concepts around this topic to further support your journey.

Go organic, where you can

Eating organically grown and reared foods can benefit your health exponentially, largely because of organic foods haven't been subject to refinement, or pumped full of chemicals and preservatives.

I'd be chronically lying if I told you I ate everything organic. It is a distant dream of mine to own a plot of land that I can farm – to do my part on mother earth and my own health. I would wholeheartedly love to make that a reality and to become 100% organic. But of course, it's both expensive and sometimes difficult to find organic alternatives to all of the food we eat. I've tried my best to incorporate organic foods into my weekly shop, but even by my standards I've only done okay.

Living in a digital age, where everything is urgent and everything is done to save time, we become imbued with the dangers of instant gratification. We have become used to it, the same way you become used to eating fast food. Take the time to find the best places to buy organic produce, budget for it and buy it when you can.

If you can't go organic, at least eat wholefoods – meat that hasn't been processed, grains that haven't been refined, food that wasn't pre-prepared in a factory. This is a great step in the right direction. And when you create your own meals and cook your own food, at least you control what goes into it.

Stay Hydrated

I cannot stress enough how important it is to stay hydrated. Human bodies are made of up to 60 percent water – and just like an indoor plant, we'll wither if we don't have enough fluids.

Drinking water during training will stop your body from becoming dehydrated. It will also aid digestion and circulation, and can help with cravings, too.

It is equally as important that you replace electrolytes after a heavy training session, and you can buy pre-bottled waters that contain the appropriate minerals. If you are on a diet and also sweating a lot, you will lose vital minerals, so replacing these is key. Again, check the label to know what you are about to consume.

Professor Gerald H Pollack is a scientist who wrote a book called *The Fourth Phase of Water* (2013). Without going into too much detail, it states that water can have a different value depending on whether it's from the tap or from a mountain stream. This is not only because of the minerals that are present, but also because of its compound structure. Water in our body's cells contains H_3O_2. When we drink water from the tap, our body has to convert it from H_2O to H_3O_2. This is otherwise known as EZ (exclusion zone) water and can be found in spring water straight from the mountains, or in watery fibrous vegetables. In this form it is also more replenishing because it has more nutrients than regular tap water. As long as you filter your water, you can ensure its quality. Bottled water is problematic as plastic bottles are single-use plastic devastation for the planet; plus studies have shown that there are plastic particles found in most bottled water. Glass bottles are the way forward if you're buying water.

Cheat meals

A note, now, about cheat meals, also known as sin food or off days. Whatever you call it and however you approach a break from your diet and training, remember: *do not punish yourself because you've eaten something you consider bad*. Don't try to starve yourself for the next week to compensate for a few extra calories consumed. One cheat meal is not going to derail your whole programme – you should only worry if that one cheat meal becomes a cheat day and then a whole cheat weekend.

Instead, if you slip, just return to your regular eating pattern, consuming good clean food. Once your body is conditioned with wholefoods, you will actually feel bad and maybe even a little sick if you consume too much sugar or lots of processed food, so there is no need to beat yourself up psychologically, as well.

Just relax and return to your plan. Cheat meals and off days are meant to be a treat or a reward for all of your hard work. With that said, if you haven't worked hard and if you're not eating healthy wholefoods to begin with, then it's not really a cheat meal, is it?

Personally, I don't factor cheat meals into my routine, but that's not to say I won't indulge every now and again, but I actually enjoy eating healthy food. I like sweet treats, but I love health way more. I don't have cheat meals every week. I can go a good few months without a treat, if I so desire, but that's down to my conditioning.

It's all about creating healthy habits, and this doesn't take as long as you might think.

For me, personally, I always ask myself what is the benefit of me eating that? And, when being healthy is fun for you, it really does become second nature.

If you find holidays, such as Christmas, tricky, the key is to make sure you have a damage prevention strategy in place – beforehand. So, rather than fighting to work off the calories afterwards, why not try prepping for the feast to come. As well as some resistance training before a big blow out, you could try:

>> **Spending at least 4 or 5 days intermittent fasting (16/8 is quite reasonable)**

>> **Drinking apple cider vinegar (*see* page 128) 1–2 times per day, or eating some fermented food**

>> **Eating lots of green leafy veg**

>> **Training in a fasted state (if in the morning)**

>> **Not eating too late**

>> **A couple of days of keto (low carb)**

>> **Black coffee / matcha tea, which are both thermogenic**

>> **Cold showers / jogging in the cold / cold water therapy**

>> **Getting quality sleep of at least 6.5 hours a night**

EATING TO PROMOTE MUSCLE GROWTH

I've actually been doing this for years. When Christmas comes and it's time to indulge, I never put on much weight because I'm already ahead of the game. I may end up consuming a lot of food but the following day I will go back to normal and maybe fit in some jogging, or some circuits and my diet will return to normal.

Rather than starving myself, I will go through a detox instead, taking activated charcoal, plus a special smoothie and some glutathione to help digest all of the extra calories I've consumed.

Break the routine

That 'R' word again. It is the patterns we form from repetitive behaviour that often have the greatest detrimental impact to our health. This might be bad food choices, such as eating at your desk or late at night. Over time, these things become habit and are then difficult to break.

If you have a hot chocolate before bed every night because that's part of your routine, imagine how that is impacting your diet. There are the added calories, the spike in insulin due to the extra sugar, and the habitual nature of doing it every day. Also consider how eating or drinking so close to bed will disrupt your sleep, forcing you to go to the toilet in the night. All of these things will impact your energy the following day.

So, take some time to think about any eating habits you need to break. But also, remember to enjoy your food. So often, people eat on autopilot, not even thinking about the food they are taking in, just stuffing their faces through boredom. Grazing on nuts or crisps or having that hot chocolate or tea before bed because it helps them to relax. Next time think about the impact this might have on your body in the long term.

Good habits and routines are where it's at. Once you've trained your mind and your body to crave good things, you will see the health benefits and soon enough, you will begin to instinctively reject things that make you feel bad.

In conclusion ...

MAKE HEALTH AND FITNESS YOUR LIFE
Yes, I go to the gym, but this is only a fraction of what I mean by "fitness". Looking after your health doesn't only mean doing all the things that are right, it means getting rid of the things that are wrong.

People don't necessarily avoid the things that they shouldn't eat, they focus on buying the things that are supposed to be good. They trust in the labelling on the package to save time.

If you respect yourself, then think about what foods you consume and any natural supplements you plan to take. Don't blindly believe in the packaging if it says naturally flavoured, low fat, high protein, etc.

Anything that needs to convince you of its health benefits is usually just a marketing ploy in my experience.

Different body types will have different relationships with certain foods, and what works for one person might not work so well for another.

The point is, we are not all the same, so in the same way that we should tailor any exercise programmes to our individual needs, it is a matter of trial and error with nutrition, but it is so worth your time working out exactly what is best for just you.

"THE ART AND SCIENCE OF CHANGING THE ENVIRONMENT AROUND YOU AND INSIDE YOU, SO YOU HAVE MORE CONTROL OVER YOUR BIOLOGY."

Dave Asprey

CHAPTER 8
BIOHACKING

Biohacking is the art of leveraging your biology in order to unlock human potential. By drawing on scientific knowledge, we can analyse and improve our genetic makeup and use this information to fine-tune and optimize our approach to training and nutrition.

In this chapter, I will share with you my top biohacking tips, including grounding methods that reduce inflammation and stress, red light therapy that aids muscle recovery and function, blue light blockers, hot and cold therapies and my pick of the natural supplements available, all of which can help take your health to the next level.

How to become a biohacker 🎤

A biohacker is essentially somebody who strives to optimize their health through any practical and learned means. It's about improving your health from the cellular level up. Biohacking encompasses things that improve our wellbeing naturally and things that have been developed using modern technology. It has led me on a quest to better understand myself, whilst at the same time investigating the incredible extent of the capabilities of the human body and mind.

I've been working for many years to hack my physical and mental capabilities. Training at different times to see what feels better, adding reps, dropping sets or whatever system seems right. I've tried different types of learning modalities and I've looked at sleep tracking and monitoring myself after eating certain foods. And I regularly evaluate my mental status after facing certain stresses in my day.

Biohacking means we can take health into our own hands and use a bespoke range of remedies just for us, bettering our health through medicinal foods and cutting edge technology. Let's take a look.

Practice grounding

Do you take vitamin G? That's right, "G", it wasn't a typo. Grounding or earthing is a connection to the planet and to nature. To some, this will sound strange and you might think I've turned into a tree-hugging activist, but if you take a moment to read this it might all make sense.

Grounding: the act of removing your shoes and walking / standing / lying on a natural surface, not plastic or rubber – perhaps a short walk barefoot in your garden or on wooden floors every day will suffice. It restores our body's natural electrical stability and rhythms, which in turn promotes optimal functioning of our bodily systems including the cardiovascular, respiratory, digestive and immune systems. It also helps to reduce inflammation, which is a common cause of disease.

At home, I use a grounding mat which can measure the electrical charges that travel through the body. We are conductors for EMFs (Electric and Magnetic Fields) which creates free radicals in the body.

Studies have shown that grounding can also help you sleep better because it helps your body return to its normal electrical state, allowing us to become more efficient at self-regulating and healing.

The great thing about grounding is that it's FREE. You can purchase devices for your household (I've added some in the Resources section at the back of the book), to maximise your grounding experience and enable you to do it indoors, but you don't have to. You can also utilize your local surroundings to achieve these effects, too.

Every morning, I spend some time outside walking barefoot on the grass. This form of earthing allows me to reconnect with the earth's natural energies and re-energize myself.

This kind of natural grounding is why people feel great when they spend time overseas in warmer climates. Your feet are exposed when you walk on the beach, or beside the pool. This helps expel negative ions while also exposing you to the elements, meaning fresh air and vitamin D, the sunshine vitamin.

GROUNDING BY THE SEA

We connect electronically to the earth. That negative charge powered through the ground can give our cells a massive boost, so being barefoot as often as possible is hugely beneficial. So, why do we feel so great when we're by the sea? The sun is the most bio-available way to get vitamin D. If you notice you're feeling happier, it's actually because the sun increases serotonin as well, and this leads to a feeling of wellbeing and happiness.

More sunlight means a better circadian rhythm. Your body clock will thank you for it. This will make you want to back flip out of bed rather than the traditional long sigh as you lean forward to get up. The sun has an invisible ray of infrared light too. This, along with the nice heat, will detoxify your body, purify your skin, boost mitochondria and strengthen your immune system.

VITAMIN D AND COVID-19

Vitamin D aids bone and muscle health and is particularly beneficial to those at high risk from COVID-19. Research has shown that the combination of vitamin K_2 & vitamin D3 is more effective in preventing bone loss than either nutrient alone.

Red light therapy 🎙️

Red light therapy (RLT) is a treatment whereby you expose yourself to low levels of red or near-infrared light. Infrared light is a type of energy that your eyes can't see, but your body can feel as heat – much of the sun's energy is infrared. Red light, such as that given off by a red light panel that you can buy, is similar to infrared, but you can see it. Red light is said to be extremely beneficial for improving health on both a superficial and cellular level. Some of its benefits include:

>> **Reducing wrinkles and improving collagen**
>> **Boosting of mitochondrial health**
>> **Muscle recovery**
>> **Deeper REM sleep**
>> **Elevation of testosterone and sex drive**

Red light helps to strengthen and boost your mitochondria (*see* page 124), helps to boost collagen within the skin and can help remove scarring. It can also help to wake you up, as it imitates the light spectrum we get from natural daylight. As the sun begins to rise, it omits red light – the awakening light. The spectrum changes later in the afternoon and turns to blue, which aids alertness.

I will use a red light panel as a boost before I go to the gym.

Red light panels come in different sizes, different models; anything from a full-body panels to smaller handheld devices. These can even help to boost testosterone, which helps to retain muscle, especially in older men.

Exposure to the sun works as a natural alternative to RLT. Infrared light helps us on a cellular level, producing ATP (adenosine triphosphate) in mitochondria. This is why I spend so much time outside, exposing as much skin as possible to natural light. It's good for boosting endorphins, too.

Blue light

Our bodies operate a circadian rhythm, which is essentially our internal body clock that tells us when to sleep and when to wake up.

The sun produces blue light helps with alertness. It helps with memory and cognitive function, as well. That's why, when it's sunny our mood is boosted and we feel alert and ready to start our day. When the sun goes down, the blue light disappears and our circadian rhythm informs us that it's time to go to bed. Soon enough, we begin to feel tired because our melatonin levels have increased.

Many of our screens and digital devices emit blue light. What many people don't realize is that sitting on the sofa or in bed on your phone not only affects your circadian rhythm (affecting REM sleep) but it can also affect the DHA (Docosahexaenoic acid) in your eyes.

Additionally, blue light emitted from LED screens, such as computers, phones and televisions has been proven to disrupt sleep and is thought to be a cause of insomnia, mood and a lack of concentration.

Sleep is one of the fundamentals for a healthier, longer life. Good sleep detoxes the brain and will set you up for the following day. It also aids the stimulation of testosterone and HGH, as well. The more REM and deep sleep we have, the better our wellbeing. People who deprive themselves of quality sleep on a regular basis pay later on, not only from their loss in productivity but it also unlocks doors to dementia, Type 2 diabetes, weight (fat) gain and a whole host of other problems. So, if you spend several hours a day in front of an LED screen with artificial blue light then be smart and do something about it.

Blue light blockers are glasses that filter blue light and are a great biohacking tool. You can also purchase apps that filter blue / green wavelengths, though the best and most natural way to prevent blue light is to avoid looking at screens before bed.

WHAT ARE MITOCHONDRIA?

Mitochondria are the parts of our cells responsible for energy production – they are known as the powerhouses of our cells. They produce energy-carrying molecules called ATP which release fuel after the breakdown of food.

More often than not, cognitive decline occurs because of external factors such as stress, or by inhibiting of certain foods and things that we consume on a regular basis. If you don't eat well, you can't think well – it's that simple. When dopamine and serotonin rise after the consumption of sugary foods, the body takes a mental nose dive, as does your mitochondria.

Time restricted eating (*see* page 98) also stimulates AMPK (AMP-activated protein kinase). This is like a regulator of energy homeostasis. If you want more ATP from your powerhouse mitochondria which increases fat oxidation, glucose uptake and fat utilisation, then this is the way forward.

Hot and cold therapies

The use of hot and cold treatments, including ice baths and saunas, can play a part in rehabilitating injuries and alleviating pain in aching muscles and joints, and I use them regularly. They can also be a great way to relax or reinvigorate yourself.

Cold treatments help to reduce inflammation and swelling by decreasing blood flow to an injury or affected area. Heat treatments help promote blood flow and allows the muscles to relax. Heat can be used to aid chronic pain while the sauna can help alleviate stiff joints while hot stones can help remove stress from the body.

Alternating both hot and cold therapies (for example, moving from the ice bath to the sauna, and back again) may help reduce exercise-induced muscle pain. Remember, to ensure you do not expose yourself to extreme heat, and never put ice directly onto the skin.

Supplements 🎙️

If you are receiving the full nutrition from the food you eat, you should in theory not need supplements. However, lots of fancy marketing has led the general public to think that drinking whey protein is going to magically promote muscle growth.

The whey protein market is a minefield, and there are so many variants. If you do choose to use then, ensure you do your homework before buying anything. If you don't know what's in it, don't buy it.

All of the nutritional benefits of a supplement can be found in regular food, so I rarely take protein powders. I may occasionally use organic whey protein, but first I make sure my diet is full of whole foods that fulfil all of my nutritional needs.

Digestive Enzymes are something I do recommend (*see* page 110). These aid digestion by breaking down macromolecules, helping the body to better absorb food and use it as fuel.

kApex is something I take that aids the breakdown of fat as energy. This is really good if like me you are following a ketogenic diet.

Masszymes contains protease which assists in the breakdown of protien into smaller amino acids which the body can use for energy.

Gluten Guardian is another digestive enzyme I take that helps the body break down gluten, starches and sugars.

Other simple ingredients (often found in whey powder) that I do think are beneficial in single supplement form include:

Magnesium Breakthrough is a formula that aids digestion and sleep. Magesium also helps regulate blood sugar levels and muscle function.

Zinc is great for testosterone support.

L carnatine shuttles fat into the mitochondria aiding energy production.

Primergen is a multivitamin complex in liquid form which has a significantly higher absorption rate in the body.

HRW (hydrogen water). Studies have shown that hydrogen water can help with the reduction of oxidative stress.

Water I cannot stress enough the importance of hydration.

Colostrum is something I recently discovered and is an important source of nutrients and the health benefits are astronomical; it promotes growth and fights disease in infants, but it can also be consumed during other phases of life, in supplement form, to aid immunity, help fight infection, and improve gut health.

Colostrum is the milky liquid that's released by mammals that have recently given birth, before breast milk production begins. It contains more nutrients than regular milk and also contains a chymosin coating which ensures the nutrients are delivered to the gut intact, thereby increasing its bio-availability (the ability for it to be effectively absorbed by your body). This basically means that in a natural state our gut acid destroys certain nutrients and we lose out on many benefits as a result. Consuming a supplement of dried colostrum will aid the absorption of nutrients, which has many health benefits.

The bad news is if you're vegan then you'll have to strike this off your shopping list, but the good news is that it's available in dried, raw form with no manipulation and is gluten-free. It is also organic, so it won't have any GMO, pesticide or hormones. If you want to maximise your health and are not squeamish, then I highly recommend trying it.

MCT oil is a supplement made from medium-chain triglyceride molecules, which are a type of fat found in coconut oil and palm oil. It is best sourced from coconut oil for its health benefits, and of course, palm oil is detrimental to the environment (unless grown sustainably) so is best avoided altogether.

MCT oil contains naturally occurring fatty acids, and it is used mainly by fitness professionals for its ability to produce ketones in the blood, enabling the body to utilize fat as energy (*see* page 91–2).

It is known to promote the hormone leptin, which is responsible for satiety, so it can help curb hunger and cravings for a longer period of time. MCT oil also supports healthy gut bacteria, which is always a good thing. Unlike other fats, it gets used immediately as energy by the body, going directly from the gut to the liver and straight to work.

As well as adding it to drinks – protein shakes, smoothies or even coffee – you can also cook with it, in the same way as regular coconut oil, if you wish. MCT oil isn't cheap though, so I would recommend using it sparingly along with other good oils. It doesn't have much of a smell, so you won't get the same aroma as regular coconut oil.

The now famous "bulletproof coffee", the energizing keto-friendly coffee where you add a dollop of high-quality butter or ghee, also uses MCT oil as one of its main ingredients and this can be a great way to get your body into a ketogenic state.

APPLE CIDER VINEGAR

Research suggests that taking apple cider vinegar may have many health benefits, including aiding digestion, lowering blood sugar, improving metabolism, burning fat and also suppressing appetite.

Organic, unfiltered apple cider vinegar also contains a substance called "the mother", which consists of strands of proteins, enzymes and friendly bacteria that give the product a murky appearance and is also beneficial to health. You can use a splash of it in soups and bone broth, or use it as the base of a salad dressing. Or, it can be mixed with water or juice.

This acid in apple cider vinegar is also effective against several types of bacteria and acts as an antimicrobial agent.

Daily hacks

While a lot of biohacking practices involve some tech and many of the things I do on a daily basis require specialist kit, there are some simple methods and natural options that can be practised anywhere without devices or apparatus. These low-fi biohacks are still incredibly powerful and will boost your health and wellbeing greatly.

All you need is a quiet, safe space outside and, if it's a mild day, expose your skin (within reason) to natural light.

Use an app on your phone to measure your step count and work to improve this in small daily increments.

Take regular breaks from any screens.

Walk barefoot as well, if you can, to feel a connection to the earth. And remember to breathe in deeply. It's beautiful being surrounded by green and clean air.

Create a strategy and stick to it

The body is such a complex biological machine. There are no instruction, no manual. We can only improve or repair what we have through medicine, surgery, or by hacking our own biology.

So much of what we learn is discovered though trial and error. Even with the internet and the endless amounts of information we have available to us, we are still discovering new medicines, new cures, new vaccines, and developing new technologies that can aid our health and wellbeing.

I've spent a considerable amount of time trying to understand how my brain and my body work in tangent, trying to better figure out how I can function at the peak of my capabilities. I try to push past that as well, to test the limits of the human mind.

That's why I truly believe that biohacking is the way forward. It's where biology and chemistry meets, and perhaps even physics too, to some extent.

Biohacking can improve our health, focussing on all aspects of our physical and mental wellbeing, from weight loss to healing, enhanced brain function and anti-ageing practices. It is the peak of holistic discovery, where we can improve our minds and our bodies through synergy and simple daily practices that allow us to become both self sufficient and highly efficient beings. Functioning as one coherent, living organism – as intended.

All you need to do is set the rules, follow the practices daily, and remember, there is more to fitness than what you look like on the outside. What goes into your body, and what you do to improve brain health and mindfulness is just as important. If not more so.

CORE PRINCIPLE 8

DON'T BE AFRAID TO MAKE CHANGES

As humans we are forever trying to convince ourselves that the choices we've made must be the right ones, because once we've committed to something. We find it hard to accept that we might've just made the wrong decision. We don't like to admit something didn't work.

But there really is nothing wrong with saying: *This doesn't work, so what will*?

Never be afraid to move on.

If your eating window doesn't fit into your lifestyle, then adapt and change it. Likewise, train when and where you want to. If you don't want to go to the gym because you can't be bothered to work your legs and it's leg day, then change it up. Your body isn't going to punish you for working out your chest instead of your quads. It's far more beneficial to do something rather than nothing.

Even while working out and eating a strict diet, at certain level your body will plateau; you will find yourself in a position that many people call maintenance. That is just maintaining your physique in its current state. This is the stage where people tend to panic and will start buying supplements and fat burners to enhance their progress.

Before doing this, first consider if your diet is in check, or maybe it has plateaued. Perhaps it needs to be adjusted. If your body has adapted to your training regime, then perhaps you need to ramp it up, maybe by increasing the weights or introducing more food beforehand.

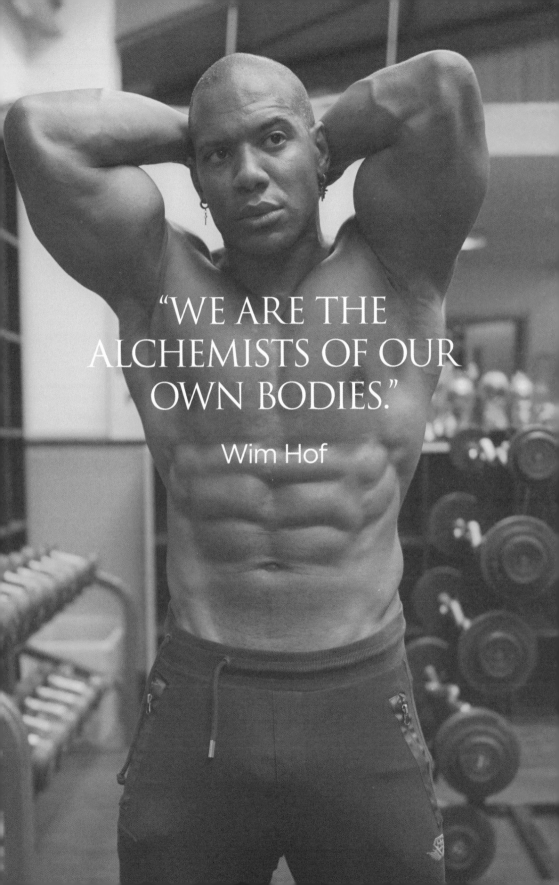

"WE ARE THE ALCHEMISTS OF OUR OWN BODIES."

Wim Hof

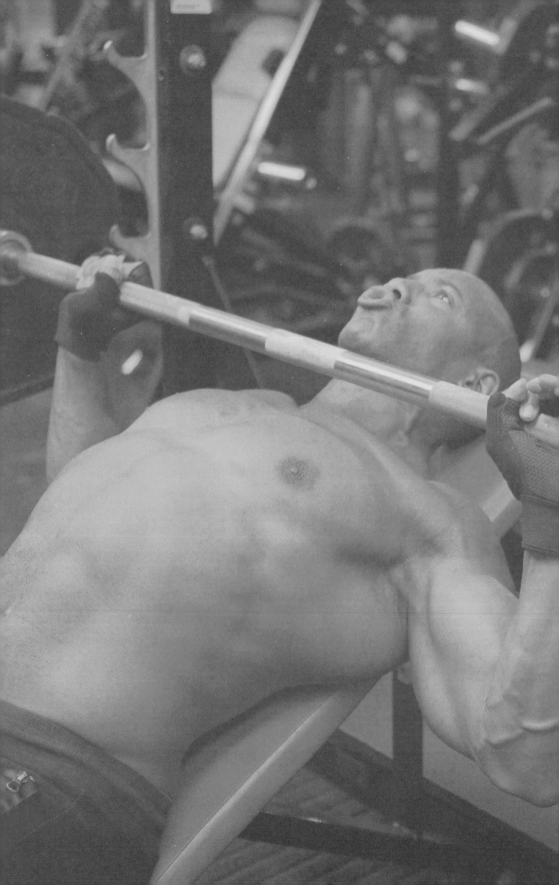

PART 4

The Roger Snipes
Workout Guide

"AS LONG AS THE
MIND CAN ENVISION
THE FACT ...
YOU CAN DO IT."

Arnold Schwarzenegger

CHAPTER 9

THE MIND-MUSCLE CONNECTION

Your mind is the MVP. Your most important asset. It drives everything. From your diet to your training regime, objectives and lifestyle – your mental wellbeing as well as your physical health. It is your most valuable asset, so take care of it and listen to it. Your mind determines how you view yourself, but it also determines how hard you work.

The mind-muscle connection, therefore, is one of the most fundamental aspects of bodybuilding training, and something that is not considered nearly enough, in my opinion, especially to those who are new to working out with weights.

In this chapter, we'll explore how to really engage your brain in your training to optimize results. We'll also take a look at some of the different ways you can train your body and aid its post-workout recovery. But let's start at the beginning – before your workout even begins – with your pre-workout state of mind.

Pre-workout

The most vital pre-workout hack is not a supplement, it's your drive.
If you don't feel the drive to work out, you'll be going into your session with failure in mind. Chances are, you'll have a half-hearted workout, or worse still, you'll end up injuring yourself. Either way, you're more likely to hinder your progress than you are to move forward.

The truth is, if you don't feel like it, then don't beat yourself up. If your drive is not there, then you need to fix this first. This desire to train needs to become ingrained, like a ritual that you must follow or a nagging voice inside your head.

Getting over that first hurdle is the hardest part. You may have to force yourself out of the door, but if you do it every day, and turn your workout into a habit, soon enough you will reverse your mood to the point where you'll be upset if you *can't* work out. Your body will crave the gym and you'll feel physically bad if you don't get exercise.

Music can be one of the best things to give you that initial bump you need and generally lift your mood. Also, having a coffee (or any type of caffeine supplement) can give you a shot of energy to get you started. Experiment with using some of the biohacks you've learned about and create yourself a pre-workout ritual that gets your head in the right place for what's to come.

AEROBIC VS ANAEROBIC EXERCISE

Aerobic and anaerobic are terms used to describe how cells within the body produce energy in opposing ways.

Aerobic means "with air". This is where the body produces energy with the use of oxygen. Aerobic exercises are usually continuous steady-state exercises, such as jogging, cycling, boxercise or general fitness classes. Essentially what we call cardio. These will get your blood flowing and your heart racing and are generally best for losing weight.

Anaerobic means "without air". This is typically exercise that is performed at a higher intensity and will incorporate explosive workouts such as HIIT or free weights. Anaerobic exercise is better for building muscle, strength and endurance.

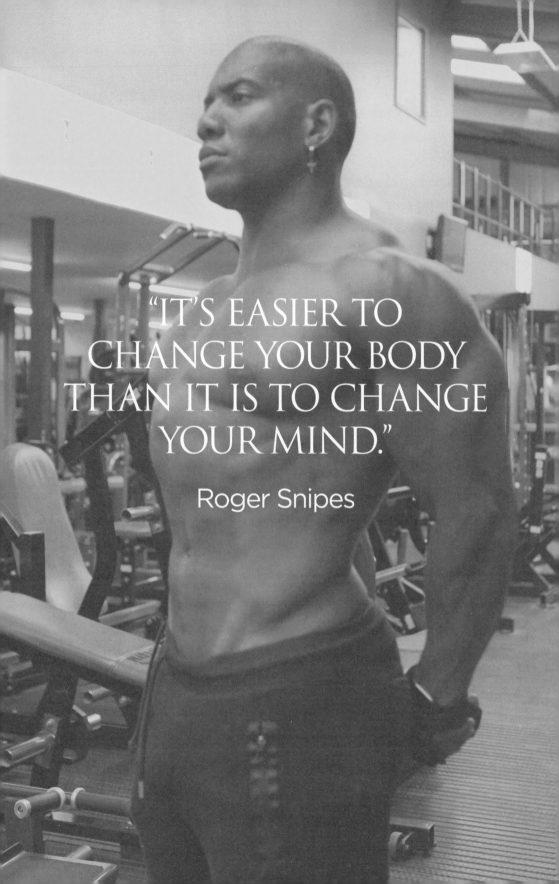

"IT'S EASIER TO CHANGE YOUR BODY THAN IT IS TO CHANGE YOUR MIND."

Roger Snipes

Train smarter

Work harder or work smarter?

As we've seen, your body is a product of your mind and, as the saying goes, you can't outwork a poor diet. With that in mind, my advice is to both work hard and work smart, but make it 80 percent smart *and* 20 percent difficult. These are my top tips for smart training:

›› **ENSURE YOUR DIET IS ALIGNED WITH YOUR TRAINING GOALS**
Your diet will determine your energy levels and most likely, will reflect your base level of fitness as well, so make sure it supports your fitness goals.

›› **START YOUR WORKOUT WITH A PLAN**
Rather than blindly performing an exercise because you've seen others doing it, or because it looks easy or effective, ensure you know exactly which muscle group you are actually hitting when you start.

›› **PICK THE CORRECT WEIGHTS FOR THE JOB**
Always consider the consequences of how you train. Lifting heavy is pointless if you don't know what muscle group you're working. If the weight is too heavy for you, you will just end up getting injured. Likewise, lifting too light will have the adverse effect and will become an aerobic exercise (*see* page 136). This will cause your body to burn fat and possibly muscle, as well.

›› **ALWAYS CHECK YOUR POSTURE AND FORM IS CORRECT FOR THE EXERCISE YOU'RE ABOUT TO DO**
When training, using the correct form and body position will deter or reduce your chances of injury. It will also help you focus your energy. If the muscle you're working is not under stress, your form is incorrect. Adjust your grip or your stance until the weight is working the muscle. If the muscle is not placed under stress, then it will not be forced to grow.

›› **BREATHE DEEPLY AND FOCUS ON SQUEEZING THE MUSCLE ON CONTRACTIONS**
This will enhance the effort and put more stress on the muscle. After several reps you should feel the blood coursing through your muscle and after a number of sets you should feel the burn.

›› **PERFORM SLOW ECCENTRICS TO STRENGTHEN MUSCLES FURTHER**
This is when you come out of each rep of an exercise *slowly*. So, in a biceps curl, it's the lowering of the dumbbell back down from the lift. An eccentric contraction is the lengthening of the muscle while it's under load. If you do this slowly, say taking 3–5 seconds each time to come out of the curl, this will help to increase the microtears and strengthen the muscles more. Eccentric contractions recruit more muscle fibres while also burning more calories.

These are all smart techniques or approaches to get the same job done – building your muscles – but doing it a lot more effectively.

CORE PRINCIPLE 9

NEVER STOP LEARNING

Some people find a training method that works for them – an exercise they like, or a diet that helps lose a little fat – and they figure that learning *why* it actually works serves little purpose. They stick with that one thing, and never consider there might be other options or tweaks that can improve it. Part of working smarter involves taking a little time to consider how the science behind something can really change your understanding of an exercise or specific diet, especially as you grow and adapt.

As your fitness levels improve, then so too will your tolerance to certain foods and training routines. Getting from 30 percent to 15 percent body fat is by no means an easy feat, but getting from 15 percent to 10 percent, or from 10 percent to 8 percent is a lot harder. The body wants to hold on to fat (and water) so we have to adapt and almost trick it into using it as fuel. This is how the ketogenic diet works (*see* pages 91–2). This is why lifting heavy weights are more effective for weight loss than, say, cardio. So many men and women avoid lifting heavy weights because they fear they will become musclebound. Others meanwhile still believe that muscle can turn to fat. Both are nonsense. A little research will go a long way.

Even while working out and eating a strict diet, at certain level your body will plateau; you will find yourself in a position that many people call maintenance. That is just maintaining your physique in its current state. This is the stage where people tend to panic and will start buying supplements and fat burners to enhance their progress.

Before doing this, first consider if your diet is in check, or maybe it has plateaued. If your body has adapted to your training regime, then perhaps you need to adjust or ramp it up, maybe by increasing the weights or introducing more food beforehand.

VISUALIZATION

Whenever I go to the gym, the first thing I do is pick up a weight and visualize the muscle group I intend to work. I visualize the blood coursing through that muscle and the connective tissue that links to it. I think about the movement. I visualize what I'm trying to achieve – which part of the muscle I'm trying to hit – and I try to feel the results as the weight shifts from one position to another.

Before you start an exercise, visualize it. If you don't feel tension in the correct place, then either you are not working hard enough, or you are not doing the exercise correctly. Adjust your position until you do. And then continue to keep your mind focused on the task in hand. Don't zone out when you work out.

Overtraining

It's never enough to give your best only some of the time. Anything worth doing is worth doing 100 percent, or you may as well save your energy and not do anything at all.

With that said, trying to give 110 percent all of the time is both impossible and is destined to failure.

In the fitness industry this is called overtraining. Unfortunately, this is a principle that many people seem to abide by – they work out excessively, spending too long in the gym, and don't allow their bodies adequate rest. Overtraining leads to a whole host of issues, such as adrenal fatigue, sore joints, damaged tendons and ligaments, not to mention torn muscles. It is not great for longevity and continued performance in the gym.

Don't overdo it. Overtraining can lead to burnout, or worse, injury. Take time off. Let your muscles rest and recover before you punish them again.

Instead, follow a regime of adopting progressive overload exercises into your workout instead. Progressive overload is the process of steadily increasing the weight and continually making your muscles work harder. This will add the necessary controlled stress to your muscles, forcing you to reach failure (where your muscles fatigue), which will in turn force them to grow.

Shake up your routine

Training is about putting your muscles under stress so that your body learns to adapt to the extra load by breaking down muscle tissues and fibres before building them back up, bigger and stronger than before.

Some people sometimes train while in a calorie deficit, and some train fasted. These approaches have different effects, which we'll look at in a moment. However, what I would always recommend is keeping an open mind and mixing things up a little so you don't ever get stale, bored or complacent in the gym.

Here are some of my top tips for keeping things fresh in your workout.

›› **Try alternating workouts.** Do free weights one day and then cardio or a HIIT the next. You could also try circuits, multiple sets, pyramid sets, drop sets, super sets or a split-routine system when you want to isolate detail in each muscle group.

›› **If you go into the gym with a plan to train a certain way but find your energy levels are down for whatever reason, give yourself permission to change on the spot.** It really is ok to do this. I'm regimented in my goals, but if I'm not feeling it or if I lack energy, then I might instead focus on some isometric contractions. These are static exercises such as plank or side bridge, where you hold a position rather than create momentum. They *maintain* muscle strength rather than build more. It is absolutely ok to do this! You don't have to continually build, in order to be strong.

Slow eccentrics is a standard procedure for me, but giving a 2, 3 or 5 second pause / hold is a good way of challenging yourself without overdoing it if you are suffering from muscle fatigue.

›› **If you're feeling stronger, you can change things up too.** Take the lifts you have planned and increase them or make them tougher. If my plan was to bench 140kg (310lb) but I was feeling great, il might do 150kg (330lb) instead and then gauge it from there. And if I was still feeling strong then I might add another 2.5kg (5.5lb) each side, at least.

›› **Try alternating location.** Mix up the place where you work out. Ideally, it's good to have a gym facility as the foundation of your training for keeping and maintaining body composition. But that doesn't mean you can't incorporate a workout at home into your routine if you're pushed for time, or even an activity, such as an indoor climbing wall or a bike ride.

›› **If the weather is nice, once in a while enjoy nature's playground.** Go to a local park and take a kettle bell or do some bodyweight circuits. And while you're there, take off your shoes and try some grounding techniques (*see* pages 120–1) as well. The combination of exercise and being outside will benefit you more than being inside a stuffy gym.

Training in a calorie deficit

If you are training while in a calorie deficit (not consuming as many calories as your body is expending in energy), you should take it steady in the gym. The problem with aggressive dieting while training is that you are forcing your body to function at a high level, much like overtraining, but with the added stress of being in a calorie deficit. This can have an adverse effect on your body, forcing you into a catabolic state, which is when muscle tissue breaks down because the muscle is essentially using itself for fuel.

Muscle needs amino acids from protein to repair and to grow, so cutting or withholding calories in this state seems somewhat counterproductive. A gradual approach to a cut is always more efficient, and needs to be done over time. Trying to rapidly reduce calorie intake can cause mental stress, and it can be physically damaging as well, especially if you're still working out at an optimal capacity on top. Chances are, if you've significantly reduced calories then you are hoping to lose body fat, which means you will most likely not want to slow down in the gym.

Alternatively, if you're trying to build muscle then you're going to have to respect your body's chemistry. This is key! Force-feeding yourself for size may indeed trigger the wrong type of hormone. Again, a gradual, moderate approach is best.

If you adopt a desperate or aggressive approach to your diet and workout – perhaps you just want to get in shape for a holiday, or maybe you're getting married in a few months, or you've signed up for a bodybuilding competition and you're slightly unprepared – then it may, of course, be possible to get down to a desired weight or attain your desired body-fat percentage. But this is not a sustainable way to achieve a good physique in the long-term.

Mentally, it takes time to reframe your approach to fitness and if you are embarking on a new fitness journey then you need to take things slowly. Don't cut calories, but instead ensure your calories are coming from good-quality food sources. If anything, you will probably find that you will need to consume more calories to sustain the heavy workouts (unless your plain is to cut weight / lose fat).

In both cases, if you eat a slight surplus of calories – perhaps just 10% kcals over your maintenance, you should be able to build lean muscle mass and create a solid frame that is not impossible to maintain.

Training fasted

However, there is evidence to suggest that training fasted – working out before you have eaten, say, first thing in the morning – can increase metabolism and growth hormone, and I would highly suggest trying a fasted workout if you are keen to lose weight while still working out to your full potential.

Training fasted allows more metabolic flexibility, which is your ability to utilize glycogen for energy more effectively while also losing body fat at the same time.

And for those of you who are pre-diabetic, this will benefit you a great deal too.

But, of course, you must make sure you sufficiently refuel your body afterwards. If you're a beginner and your body is not used to working in a fasted state, I would suggest building up a fasted training routine gradually – don't do it every day to begin with – wait until your body has fully adapted. Without sufficient fuel, your body will only be firing at a percentage of full capacity and you risk injury or burnout doing too much too soon.

Rest and recovery

Building muscle mass doesn't all happen in one go. The body needs to rest in order for reconstruction to occur. During this time the body rebuilds any damaged tissues, nutrients are replenished, the parasympathetic nervous system kicks in – this is when the body is at its best for rejuvenation and growth.

When you train, the goal is to create trauma to the muscles in the form of something called microtears. When this happens, the body will respond by learning to adapt to the situation, so it can manage the workload easier by recruiting new muscle fibres.

One essential component of rest and recovery is sleep. Nothing aids both your mind and body like it – quality sleep is when we repair. Good sleep means more energy and sharper focus for the day ahead. Your hormones will become more balanced, and you will have less chance of wanting to snack on garbage food, which will of course stop you feeling like garbage.

Sleep also impacts glucose. Stress can be caused when we lose sleep, forcing our cortisol levels to rise, which in turn raises our glucose levels. The body translates this lack of sleep as a stress. Our fight or flight response is triggered and we then produce glucose because our body thinks we require more energy. This is why sometimes we get in bed and suddenly don't feel tired.

MASSAGE

To many people, a massage is something you only have if you're a sports' professional or are physically active with some type of sports hobby. But a deep tissue sports massage, or any kind of massage for that matter, has incredible benefits and is also a great way to treat yourself, and help you relax. A good massage will rid you of unwanted stresses and may also identify areas where injuries or muscle tears are prevalent. The additional benefits of a regular massage are as follows:

›› **Increased blood flow**

›› **Reduced recovery time**

›› **Release of muscle tissue damage, knots and back pain**

›› **Better dispersal of lactic acid (see DOMS box below)**

›› **Breaking down of scar tissue**

Massage guns are also available if you don't like the thought of a stranger manhandling you. These can be bought in stores and online and can range from £50 to £700.

Find one that's well-reviewed and suits you and your budget. More expensive doesn't always mean that it's better suited for your needs.

DOMS

Delayed onset muscle soreness, or DOMS as it's more commonly known, is a deferred pain in the muscles brought on by the build-up of lactic acid, usually after a heavy workout or when an exercise has been completed without sufficient warm-up; or, more often than not, because your body is not accustomed to the stress it has been put under.

DOMS usually occurs one or two days after an intense workout and can last anything up to a week. You can't really prevent DOMS as it is a sign of your muscles recovering. But with adequate stretching before and after a workout, you can limit the amount of discomfort DOMS causes you.

HEAVY LIFTING

Lifting heavy weights will not only burn a greater number of calories and boost testosterone, but it will also increase endurance, strengthen bone structure and the skeletal muscles. Improving the skeletal muscles helps with homeostasis, which aids internal stability.

CAUTION: Always make sure you have a spot (someone to assist you), a personal trainer, coach or some other assistance when performing a heavy bench press or squats, to avoid an injury or accident.

How I stay in shape

When you're always in shape, people assume you don't make any changes to your body. This really isn't true. I'm always trying out new things – biohacks or just mixing up what I do for fitness.

This year I've taken a strong interest in cycling and intermittent fasting. My food choices are still healthy and whole, but my diet also now includes an array of micronutrients, adaptogenic herbs and holistic therapies, as well as some wild plants, to aid digestion. Alongside this, I work out between two and three times a week.

Once your body is conditioned as mine is, it requires less work, which is another benefit of building a great physique. Provided you don't abuse it, it will become a self-sufficient machine. And being in great shape affords you the freedom to try out new things, such as cycling, because you have the fitness levels to basically try out anything!

I'm definitely feeling more complete in terms of health than when I started 20+ years ago. I always have more things on my checklist that I want to research, such as the field of genes and genetic tests, telomeres tests (to measure biological age) and ancestral research. Science has taken us so far, so it's important we use it.

On a daily basis, I go by the way I feel. If I don't feel mentally there, I will spend more time on wellness. I will take additional time with the red light, or the Nano-V (see the Resources), or I use the Muse, a guided meditation which picks up the waves in my head and can detect frequency as soundwaves.

If I feel down or cold, and I don't feel like going outside, or working out, I will then push myself to go outside. I will jog without a top on, facing the thing I dread. This always makes me feel better, physically and mentally. It gets the blood pumping – I soon forget the cold and have such a sense of achievement when I'm done that it's always worth it.

In a sense, this is what we do in the gym. We should challenge ourselves to face things that might make us a little uncomfortable, because this is how we get stronger. Don't be tempted to try too much, too soon, but pushing yourself just a little more each time is how we provoke change.

So you can see that, it really is about how your mind builds your body. Getting your head in the right space is key for a successful workout, but you also need to use your head when considering the best nutrition to power your body, while all the time remembering to take care of yourself mentally. Treat your fitness journey holistically to get the best and most long-lasting results.

CHAPTER 10

TRAINING FUNDAMENTALS

In this chapter, you will find a comprehensive plan of simple but effective core exercises. Together with the positive mental approach, nutrition and biohacking techniques we have explored elsewhere in this book, these will enable you to build a solid foundation that will put you beyond the run-of-the-mill gym goer.

I will give you key workout exercises and form tips for each major body part, as well as providing variations or alternative exercises in case you are unable to perform the one that has been outlined for any reason.

There are six body areas covered (legs, chest, back, core, arms and shoulders). Consider this an exercise buffet. Pick and choose from the exercises here, and create a workout plan that suits your body, time, and energy levels. Mix and match them each time you work out, or build a familiar pattern with repeating the same workout for three weeks at a time. It is UP TO YOU. If you feel your body plateauing, change it up and focus on different exercises.

Let's start with the all-important warm-up stretches that should be done before undertaking any rigorous form of exercise, particularly when lifting heavy weights.

WARM-UPS

It is vital that you warm-up all necessary body parts before vigorous exercise and using free weights. This should be done with a combination of controlled isolated stretches and some light cardio work such as jumping jacks or burpees, to fire up the respiratory system. Do each of the following stretches at least once, breathing deeply, to thoroughly warm-up your body before your workout.

Child's pose, extended

This is a yoga stretch, good for relaxing the shoulders and stretching the lower back.

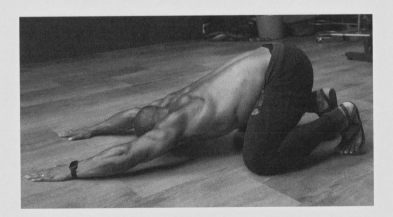

HOW TO PERFORM THIS EXERCISE
Kneeling down, place your hands flat on the floor stretched out in front of you, rest your forehead on the floor, push your chest toward the ground and hold for a few breaths.

Triceps / above the head chest stretch

HOW TO PERFORM THIS EXERCISE

1 Lift your left elbow above the shoulder and push back on it with your other hand while reaching your left hand down the centre of your back. This will stretch out your triceps, shoulders and your neck.

2 Hold for 10 to 15 seconds, then repeat with the other arm.

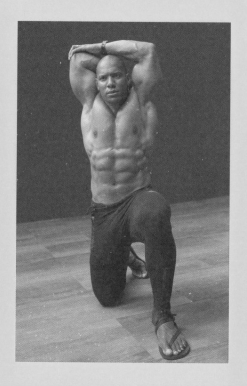

Behind the back wrist-grip / shoulder squeeze

This stretch is good for the arms, shoulders back and chest.

HOW TO PERFORM THIS EXERCISE

1 Move your arms behind your back and hold one wrist with the opposite hand.

2 Move the position of your grip to engage different muscles and hold the pose for 10 seconds, then release. Repeat.

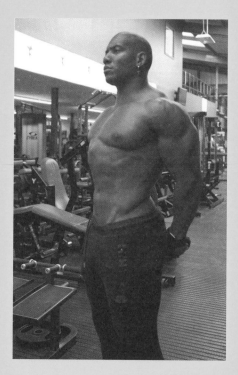

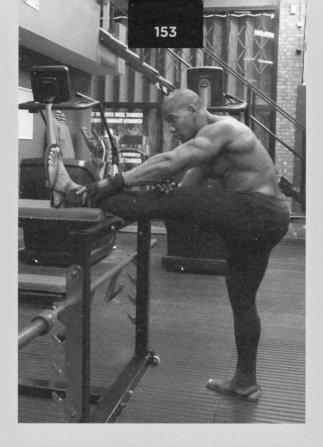

Hamstring stretches

This is a standard, go-to stretch that you should do before any leg training. The key here is balance.

**HOW TO PERFORM
THIS EXERCISE**

1 Place one leg horizontally out in front of you so it rests on a sturdy level surface. Ensure the leg is straight, with the other leg slightly bent and your foot at a 45-degree angle.

2 Without rocking or bouncing, lean forward with your hands and hold onto (or as near to) your ankle as you can.

3 Do this 10 times and hold for 20 seconds each time, and then repeat with the other leg.

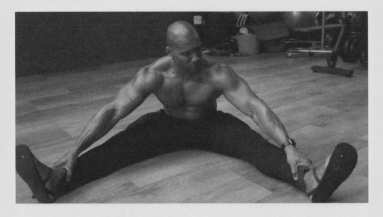

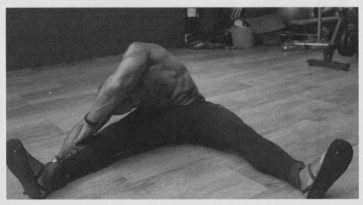

Straddle stretch / seated split

HOW TO PERFORM
THIS EXERCISE

1 Sit on the floor with your legs as wide apart as is comfortable.

2 As with the hamstring stretch, extend your hands toward your ankle on either side of one leg and hold. This will stretch the inner thigh, the hips and also the hamstrings.

3 Do this 10 times and hold for 20 seconds each time, and then repeat with the other leg.

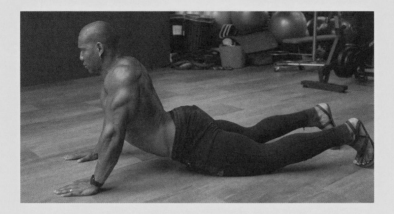

Cobra pose

This stretch opens the upper body. Make sure you don't compress the lower back.

HOW TO PERFORM THIS EXERCISE

1 Lying on your front, place your hands shoulder width apart and push upward, keeping your arms straight with your hips pushed to the floor.

2 Remember to keep your head up and your eyes straight ahead. Take 5 long deep breaths, then relax down.

WEIGHT TRAINING – SETS AND REPS

With all of the exercises that follow, I recommend performing between 8 and 12 repetitions, and between 3 and 5 sets for each exercise, depending on the weight.

Lighter weights mean more reps can be performed and more sets; with heavier weights, do fewer reps and sets, with more rest time in between. Always take between 30 and 60 seconds rest in between each set.

COMPOUND LIFTS

Building an aesthetic body takes patience and hard work, and exactly what and how you train will depend on your overall goal. But whether you are trying to build strength, gain muscle or lose weight, there are certain fundamental exercises that should be incorporated into your training – compound lifts.

Compound lifts are considered the bread and butter of bodybuilding and I personally recommend them over any other exercise. This is because they incorporate more than one muscle group and are, therefore, incredibly efficient.

Isolation exercises, on the other hand, tend to engage one single muscle group. These are great for targeting and fine-tuning single muscle groups, but compound lifts get better overall results. Not only do they recruit a lot more muscle fibre, but the moves are very natural too. Compound lifts often engage the core and entire musculoskeletal frame, meaning that they are great at building both muscle and strength.

Some examples of compound lifts include:

>> The squat
>> Deadlifts
>> Bench press
>> Clean and press
>> Pull-ups
>> Bent-over row
>> Military press

LEG EXERCISES
(QUADS, HAMSTRINGS AND CALVES)

Training your legs is essentially the foundation of aesthetics, but they are also the muscle group that many people tend to skip.

And let's be real. Training legs is often brutal. It can make you question whether you even like training at all, and the DOMS can be unbearable! Most of us – and especially those living in colder climates such as the UK – wear trousers for most of the year, so our legs are rarely on display anyway.

But if you're thinking you might skip your legs workout, I would seriously urge you to reconsider. Experiments carried out by the *European Journal of Applied Physiology and Occupational Physiology* suggest that heavy resistance exercise (squats in this case) generate an increase in HGH and testosterone in men, meaning that training your legs, especially at an age where your T-levels are starting to decline, can be hugely beneficial for turning back the clock. And an increase in testosterone and growth hormone will support the building of muscle all over.

Training your legs should be your number one priority and if you skip leg day you are missing an opportunity.

To start my week, I generally hit my legs first, because it makes the rest of the week pale by comparison. If you're anything like me, you will also have accumulated more calories over the weekend, so this would be the ideal opportunity to burn them off.

Whenever you decide to workout, and whatever exercises you do, skip legs at your peril.

Barbell squat

The great things about squats is they can be done in so many different ways, meaning they are a great exercise to incorporate into your routine if you like variation. Bodyweight squats can be done at home, outside, in hotels rooms or on the beach. You can perform bodyweight squats with a weight (the goblet squat), as jump squats, resistance band squats, and also with kettle bells or a single weight clutched to your chest.

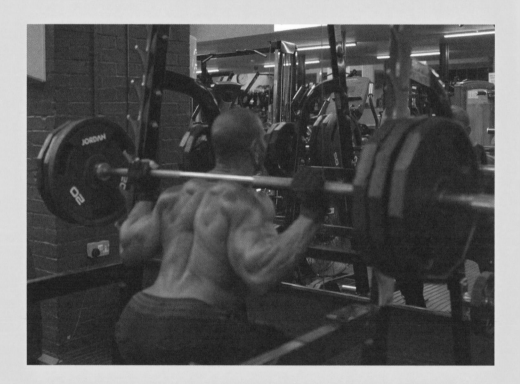

Squats can be done the old-fashioned way, too – in the gym at the squat rack where the bar is already set high so all you need to do is load the plates on, step beneath and position yourself correctly. This then allows you to lift much heavier weight than if you were lifting straight from the floor.

HOW TO PERFORM THIS EXERCISE

1 Carefully lift the bar from the rack and position it across your shoulders and traps, gripping it there with both hands. Ensure that your feet are positioned correctly – shoulder-width apart with your knees bent and your back straight.

2 Move into a sitting motion, engaging your quads and glutes. As you perform this exercise, the bar should remain in line with your feet as your knees bend and your backside goes down towards the floor. Get someone to spot you if you are unsure or are attempting to increase your lift.

3 If you have any knee issues, make sure you do not rack the weight too heavy and don't sit so low on the drop. You don't need to sit on your heels (and you can use a stool or block under your heels, if this alleviates the stress). The key is to ensure your back remains straight and your quads are engaged when you push through the floor.

The squat can be a tricky exercise to perfect because it relies so heavily on form. Dealing with the weight that you are shifting requires correct foot placement coupled with your body being in alignment and, of course, you should be thinking about the muscles you are hitting (or not quite hitting).

If you struggle to engage the muscle and lift the weight, try elevating your heels slightly (perhaps 20–30 degrees), using a piece of wood or even some smaller weight plates. This should place a greater emphasis on the quads because of the angle. The aim is to still push down on your heels, although your body weight will shift toward your toes slightly.

As a guideline, as with all of the exercises, you should attempt to do 3–5 sets of 8–12 reps.

ALTERNATIVE LEG EXERCISES

Hack squats

These are an amazing exercise if you want to primarily target the quadriceps. Hack squats can be performed with a barbell, or using a hack squat machine.

HOW TO PERFORM THIS EXERCISE

1 Using a barbell, begin with it on the floor behind you with the bar in line with your Achilles. Squat down, as if you intend to sit just above the bar, then, gripping it with both hands, slowly stand up bringing the barbell up just behind your hamstrings. Keep the torso upright while standing, squatting and coming back up.

2 Remember to breathe as you move: with the most effort on the exhalation.

Leg press

As with the hack squat, using the leg press (right) is a great exercise because the machine allows you to sit and focus solely on working the muscle.

HOW TO PERFORM THIS EXERCISE

1 This exercise is performed using a machine which mimics the range of motion of a regular (or barbell) squat – placing stress onto the quad muscles and also engaging the glutes and hamstrings. Begin with your legs bent and your knees in front of you, then extend your legs.

2 Push the plate down, but do not straighten your legs completely. Adjust your feet on the plate to hit different areas.

The leg press machine has the added benefit of putting you in a seated position to begin with, and therefore, without the added stress placed upon your neck, shoulders and back from the bar.

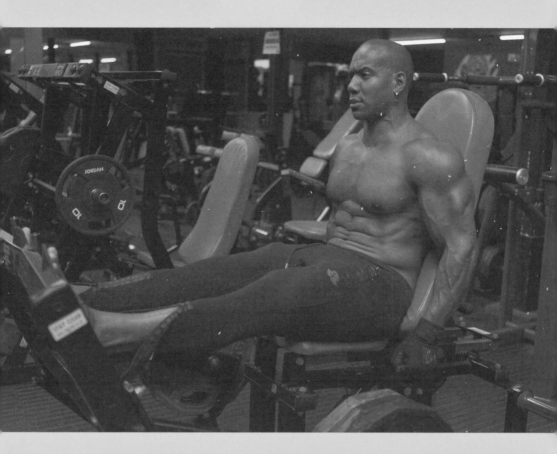

Calf press

The leg press machine (above) is also one of the few machines in the gym that allows you to work your calf muscles as well.

**HOW TO PERFORM
THIS EXERCISE**

1 Place your toes on the bottom edge of the plate, with your legs straight (but do not lock out your knees).

2 Press through your ankles to push the plate away from you with the balls of your feet. As you release the weight, your feet will bend through the ankles and your calves will stretch until you push up again for the next rep.

CHEST EXERCISES
(PECTORALS)

The chest is the centrepiece of your physique, so it's little wonder that many people covet the pec slab. Building a set of impressive pectorals is not easy, and unless you're genetically blessed with good definition and / or size, it can be one of the most difficult and frustrating muscle groups to build.

I would highly recommend the cable fly, which is a great piece of equipment for toning and teasing out those muscle striations. If size is what you want, then it may be best to persevere with the bread and butter of chest training: the bench.

Barbell bench press

The bench can be one of the most intimidating pieces of kit in the gym, and the barbell bench press can often seem to be done more for bragging rights than for actual progress. At least, that's how it feels in many of the gyms I've been to. I'm not the biggest fan of the standard bench press, to be fair, but I still do it occasionally, as done correctly it is an excellent exercise for opening up the pectorals and building a thick chest. It's definitely a great beginners' exercise for creating size and strength, provided you don't go too heavy too fast.

HOW TO PERFORM THIS EXERCISE
1 When performing the bench press, ensure your back is flat on the bench, and make sure your weight is distributed evenly. To begin with, the bar should be in line with your shoulders and, with your elbows bent, you should be able to grip it comfortably with your palms facing up and your fingers wrapped around it. As you lift the weight off the frame, hold it straight above you for a second and then bring it down

in line with your chest. Lowering the weight should take about twice as long as raising it.

2 If you struggle to bring the bar down without resting it on your chest, then the weight is probably too heavy for you. If the bar flies off with ease, then it's too light. The appropriate weight should put enough strain on your chest and shoulders to make the exercise difficult, but not impossible.

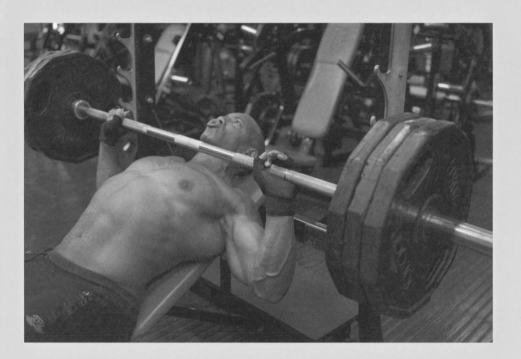

3 Ensure that you focus on pushing the bar using your chest muscles, and that you contract your pecs at the top of the controlled movement. Exhale as you push the bar up and then again as you slowly ease it down.

Remember to get someone to spot you, if you are not confident lifting the weight by yourself.

TRAINING FUNDAMENTALS

ALTERNATIVE CHEST EXERCISES

Dumbbell bench press

This is a great alternative and can be slightly less intimidating than the barbell press. It is also ideal if you suffer from shoulder injuries, as you have more freedom of movement with your grip.

The exercise is exactly the same as the barbell bench press, but with a different starting position (beginning with your weights on the floor). As you transition to heavier weights, it can sometimes be tricky to get the weight up into starting position, so ensure you train with a partner until you are strong enough to get the dumbbells into position.

Cable fly

This is an isolation exercise that will refine upper and lower chest muscles. It is great for adding detail and definition, working on those feathers and striations. Stand in the middle of the cable machine and grab each handle before placing one foot in front of the other (as though you have just taken a stride forward). Lean forward a little and slightly arch your chest forward before pushing your hands together, keeping a slight bend in your elbows, so that your hands come in front of your body just below the chest.

Hammer Strength Machine chest press

This is a solid alternative for strength and building a big, thick chest. Keep your elbows down and push the bars up at a 45-degree angle, exhaling as you do so. Ensure your elbows are pointing down as you come back down and make sure your muscles are always under tension.

Resistance push-ups (with band)

These are a great alternative if you are working out at home, or outside. Resistance bands are inexpensive and can also be carried easily in luggage. Simply, tie the band so it's one big loop and get into a push-up position. Ensure the band is across the upper part of your back while you hold it under each hand. Using the band will make the exercise a little harder at the top of the movement (holding yourself off of the ground), as the band will be resisting your upward push.

BACK EXERCISES

(TRAPS, LATS, RHOMBOIDS AND LEVATOR SCAPULAE)

The back has one of the most complex systems of interconnected muscles in the body, so it's important that before you begin working it, you warm up and stretch correctly. Also, your back is one of the most painful areas to injure – pulling a back muscle can put you out of action for a long time, so if you feel any type of twinge or strain, lay off of the weights and rest. If the pain persists, see a doctor.

Back pain is no joke.

Try performing several types of stretches beforehand, to cover a range of motion, in order to adequately stretch and warm up all of the muscles in the back. The cobra pose is a great all-round back stretch (*see* page 155).

Wide-grip pull-up (or chin-up)

The wide-grip pull-up is an all-round exercise that works the shoulders and arms as well as the back. Its primary target is the latissimus dorsi (the lats), which are the largest muscles of the upper body.

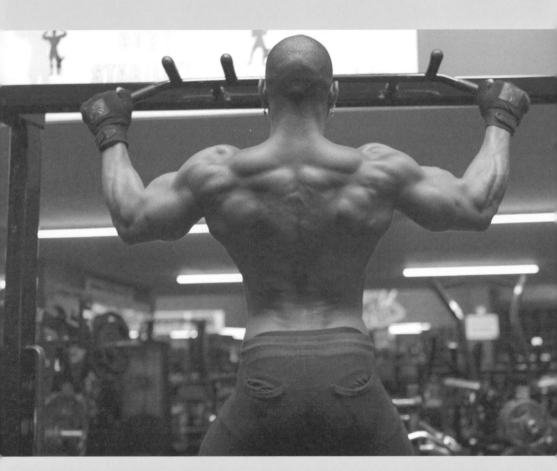

Developing big lats will give you that winger or hooded cobra look. You can perform this exercise overhand (pronated with palms facing forward) as in the image above. This is a pull-up. Alternatively, you can perform it with an underhand position (supinated with palms facing you), and this is a chin-up.

ALTERNATIVE BACK EXERCISES

A greatly developed back requires a variety of exercises. Here are a few to get you started.

Deadlift

Probably the most complete exercise in the gym. Executing every major muscle group. Just be sure to perform this one carefully, as it is easy to jar your back or neck.

Seated row

This is an awesome exercise, which will help develop the thickness and depth of the back with a strong focus on the rhomboid muscle.

Bent over barbell row

This is a great exercise for the lats and rhomboids. The position of the row allows you to build strength in the core, too.

Renegade row

As well as targeting the lats and biceps, this exercise also requires a great amount of core strength to perform it.

CORE EXERCISES

(ABDOMINALS, OBLIQUES)

Many people just focus on their abs and not the core, often believing these are the same thing. This is not the case. The core comprises two muscle types: the stabilizers and the movers, and these encompass the abdominals, the hips, the pelvis and the lower spine. There are somewhere in the region of 35 different smaller muscle groups working together. This is why people put so much emphasis on building a strong core. Having a strong core improves posture, creates stability, protects vital organs and makes you look good, and if you focus on your core the abs will follow.

Hanging leg raises

These are trickier than they might look and require a lot of upper body strength to perform, but when done correctly they will engage the entire core. The set-up is not dissimilar to a wide-grip pull-up and can be performed using the same apparatus, or on a regular straight bar. It can even be done on a strong tree branch, if you happen to be outside.

HOW TO PERFORM THIS EXERCISE

1 The key is to hang (as the name suggests) and don't be tempted to bring your arms into the exercise – they are there for stability only.

2 Keep your upper body vertical and, with your ankles held together and your legs straight, bring your feet up in front of you at 90 degrees.

3 Hold them there for a 10 count, as if you are sitting straight legged, and then slowly bring them down again.

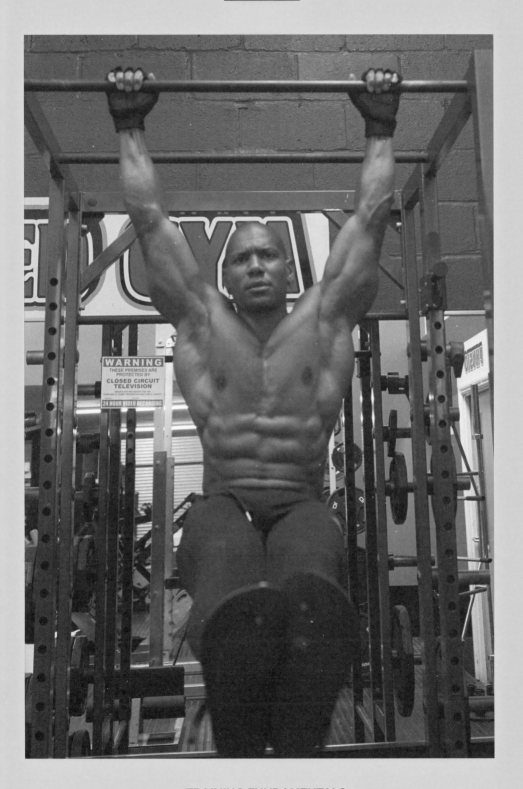

TRAINING FUNDAMENTALS

ALTERNATIVE CORE EXERCISES

Hanging knee raise

This is an alternative to the hanging leg raise and is set up in much the same way. But instead of lifting your legs straight out in front of you, the hanging knee raise allows you to bend your knees and raise them to your chest, with much the same function as a simple abdominal crunch.

Lying knee raise

These are performed lying down on the floor with your hands palm-side down by your sides. Keeping your back flush to the floor, bring your legs up in front of you with your ankles together, bending the knees. Bring your knees toward your chest before gently straightening and lowering your legs back down to the floor.

Strict toes to bar

If you are incredibly flexible, you can try the more advanced strict toes to bar exercise which involves you hanging from a bar by your hands and bringing your legs up straight in front of you. Keep going and lift them all the way up so that your toes touch the bar before lowering them down again.

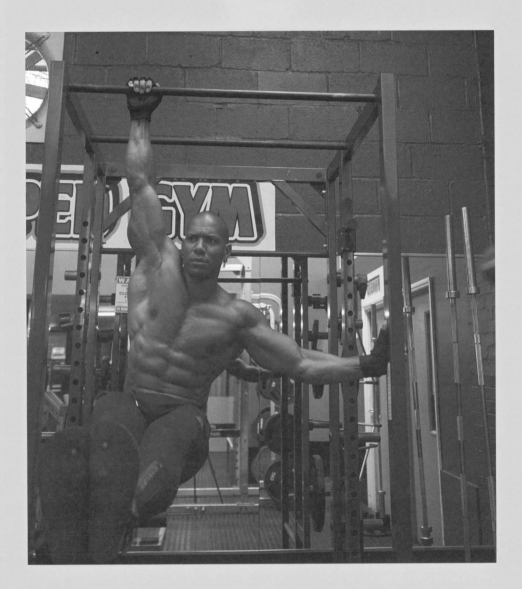

One-handed hanging leg raises

This is another variation of the hanging leg raise and one that requires great stability, using your free hand to help balance and hold yourself in place. Again, this is an advanced variation so should only be done once you have mastered the hanging leg raise. Alternate left and right arms for your sets.

ARM EXERCISES

(BICEPS, TRICEPS)

If your chest is the centrepiece of your physique, then your arms are the garnish. Many of the exercises that I've covered already incorporate arms by default. And this is why arms really do not need to be worked as often as many other body parts.

It's strange, then, that so many men focus only on their arms. Huge arm muscles – much like small legs – make you look out of proportion and this only draws attention to the areas where you need work. Your arms are already involved in virtually every upper body exercise that you do, plus they are also one of the smallest muscle groups in the body, so they don't need as much attention.

Sometimes, I only focus on biceps and skip triceps altogether, because they are now big enough. Realistically, you don't need to work your arms any more than once a week. With that said, here are some of the arm exercises that I swear by.

BICEPS

Dumbbell curls

These are probably the most common exercises you will see performed in any and every gym all over the world, with the reason being they are super effective at building up the biceps and can be performed at home if you have a simple set of weights. There are several different kinds of bicep dumbbell curls to try, and they can also be performed using a barbell to hit both biceps at once.

Unilateral exercises like the **SINGLE ARM CURL** allow you to focus on individual body parts in a bid to even out imbalances, so are a great addition to any training plan.

HOW TO PERFORM THIS EXERCISE

1 Ensure you do not swing the dumbbell; instead, tuck your elbow into your hip and slowly lower and then raise the dumbbell.

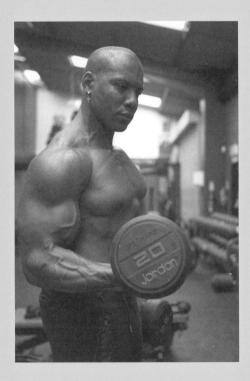 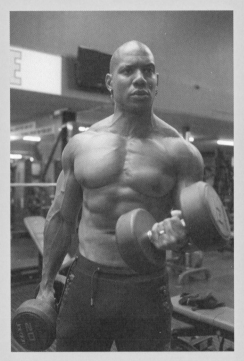

2 Make sure you get a good range of motion.

3 By changing the angle of the dumbbell slightly, you can shift focus onto either the long or short heads of the bicep. If you rotate the outside plate toward you 45 degrees you can change things up with a hammer curl.

TRAINING FUNDAMENTALS

THE CABLE CURL is another isolation exercise that focuses on the bicep muscle, which is held under constant tension. When performing a cable curl (see images below), be sure to get your grip right before you begin and lean back ever so slightly, so not to bring your back into the exercise. Ensure the arms bend only at the elbow.

This is a great exercise for beginners, or for those looking to work at high reps. It can also be performed with a single arm using a handle or D-ring attached to the cable instead of a bar.

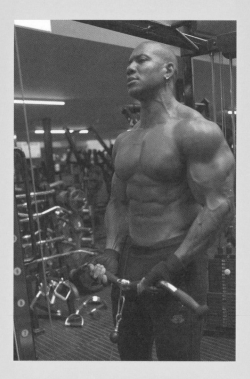
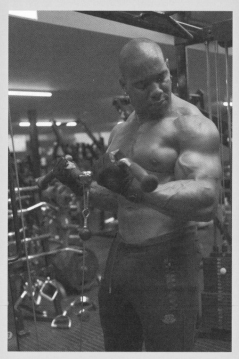

CONCENTRATION CURLS are performed dumbells and are good for the short head of the bicep and can really induce a pump. Curling the dumbell from a low hanging position, either while sitting or bending the upper body over, this creates more tension. Position your elbow just inside your knee, stabilizing your arm there. The weight essentially hangs with your arm extended (but not fully locked) out, and you bring it in toward your body, bending only the elbow as you go.

Reverse grip EZ Bar curl is a great exercise for developing the long head of the biceps so overall thickness of the arm. The motion is similar to a cable curl, only your hands are facing down – as if you're holding onto the handlebars of a bike – and then need to pull the EZ Bar up and in toward you.

Triceps

Cable rope push-down

This is an effective exercise for isolating the triceps and can be performed with a rope (right), or with a straight bar. It can be done with both arms, or by focussing on just one arm at a time.

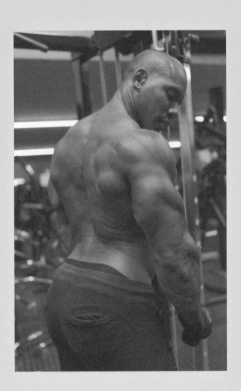

HOW TO PERFORM
THIS EXERCISE
1 Stand facing the machine, grip the rope in both hands and keep your elbows tight at your sides. Slowly force the rope downward, being careful not to hunch over or swing backward, and gradually ease off the cable to allow the rope to spring back up. Your triceps should be under constant tension for the duration of the exercise.

2 Using the cable and rope will also make it harder to force the weight when you're feeling fatigued.

Triceps kickback

This is another simple but effective exercise that will isolate the triceps.

HOW TO PERFORM THIS EXERCISE

1 Using your free hand for support, place it either on a bench or on the weight rack. Lean forward with the barbell in your free hand and set your triceps at a horizontal angle, bending your arm at the elbow like a hinge.

2 Push the weight back so your entire arm is straight, then slowly lower it, bending your arm again as you release.

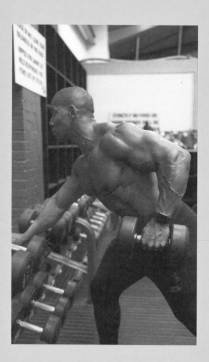 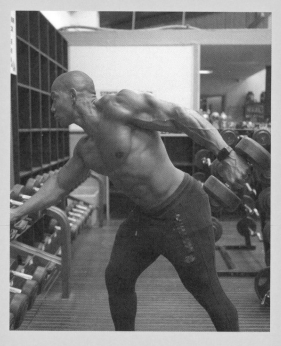

3 You should feel the tension in your triceps as you straighten your arm at the top of the move.

SHOULDER EXERCISES
(DELTOID, TRAPEZIUS)

Shoulder workouts focus primarily on the deltoids and trapezius muscles. While there are other muscles that make up the anatomy of the shoulders, these are generally the ones that get all of the praise because they are both showstoppers.

Great deltoids can appear to increase the width of one's physique and a set of boulders can give the arms that aesthetic look that many people covet. Similarly, traps can transform your appearance significantly, adding size to your entire upper body.

Military press / barbell shoulder / overhead press

Whatever you call it, this is a great compound lift that targets the deltoids, while also engaging the triceps, traps and core.

HOW TO PERFORM THIS EXERCISE

1 Your stance is important here, as is your posture. Set your feet shoulder-width apart and hold the barbell across your chest. Be careful not to lean forward and not to make any sudden jerking movements either.

2 When ready, the upward movement should be explosive but still under control. If you have to arc your head back to get the weight up, chances are it is too heavy, and you may injure yourself. Focus instead on your form.

3 I recommend beginning with a lighter weight (or even just an Olympic bar) and moving up to something a little heavier once you've mastered your form.

This exercise can also be performed with dumbbells if a barbell is not available, or alternatively with a weighted bag.

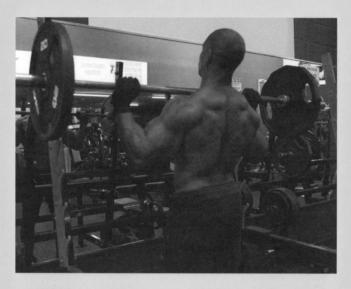

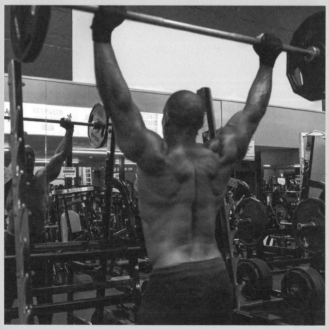

ALTERNATIVE SHOULDER EXERCISES

Lateral raises

These are an efficient isolation exercise that targets the outer head of the deltoid. Using either cables or dumbbells, grip the weights with your hands down by your sides. Keeping your arms straight, raise the weights so that they are in line with your body, pausing the lift at the top with your arms in line with your collarbone. Hold for a few seconds before slowly lowering.

Upright row

This is a great exercise to increase the size of your traps. Using either a barbell or dumbbells, this exercise is performed usually with a narrow grip on the bar, bringing it up just beneath your chin, sending your elbows in line with your ears. Again, be careful not to lean forward or rock back.

SUMMARY – MY RULES FOR SUCCESS

I follow a set of key rules to keep me focused and these are:

- ›› Food is fuel. Any pleasure I get from it is a bonus.

- ›› If it's not aligned with my goals then I'll keep away from it.

- ›› Visualize daily where I'm trying to be. This includes meditation.

- ›› Have both long-term and short-term goals for fitness.

- ›› Learn from goal setters AND go getters.

- ›› Make an opportunity from any setback. If I fall into a tub of ice cream, then I can train even harder the next day.

- ›› Training is a luxury that I am grateful for.

- ›› People respect you more if you LOOK like you respect yourself.

- ›› I'm not trying to live fast and die young. I love life.

- ›› Accountability allows me to keep on track or I'll have to make a poor excuse and led people down.

If you noticed, I didn't mention motivation. Why? Because all of these things together are what drives me.

Never rely on one rule or reason for motivation, because things can change, and that one motivating factor may not hold the strength it once did.

CONCLUSION

We all have our own dreams and fantasies, and with that, probably some idea of perfection as well.

When it comes to our own goals: how we want to look and how much we want to be liked, or like ourselves, it's human nature to want something better. But this fantasy mindset is for us and us alone, so we do not need not concern ourselves with the opinions or perceptions of others.

Recently, I was having a discussion with an elderly lady who had never left the country and she told me she had remained in the same city her entire life. She explained to me that she was very happy with her life, that she enjoyed her daily routine and did not care to travel abroad or to see anything new.

Hearing this, I was surprised. I couldn't understand why a person would be happy by not widening their horizon; having no interest in venturing out to see what the world had to offer. But, as she spoke of her choices and what she felt she had accomplished in life (raising five children being one of her many endeavours), this put things into perspective and I soon realized that I was the one with the narrow mind.

In her own way, being content to stick with a daily routine (which to me at the time seemed mundane and dreary) was an accomplishment in itself. She had found her inner happiness, and that is very rare in this world. I soon realized that she was indeed living in a fantasy world of her own making – only hers was completely different to mine.

Fantasies come in the form of dreams, goals or desires, but the main point is, they will always remain personal to the individual. What one person wants, another may fear. I now understand that I was trying to compare that lady's world with my own, and that was wrong.

Our fantasy worlds are the product of our minds. They are born out of our upbringing and our own unique experiences in life, so if we want people to be considerate of our desires, we must respect theirs, as well.

We are all different. We are all unique. Some people are happy with the way they look, and this gives them as much power as someone who has worked for years to build the perfect physique. In the end, it's all about confidence. It's all about being happy with what you see in the mirror.

The great thing for me about no longer competing is that I no longer compare myself to others. Instead, I focus on my own health – striving to become the best human being that I can possibly be – and I'm always the winner because of that mindset.

Focus should always be on your own progress, and the icing on the cake, or the butter in the coffee (only biohackers will understand that one), is when other people follow your lead.

I wish you the best of luck,

Roger Snipes

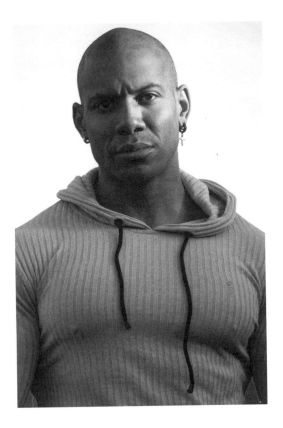

ABOUT THE AUTHOR

With more than twenty years' experience, Roger Snipes has dedicated his life and work to pushing the boundaries of human potential.

A former competitive bodybuilder and personal trainer, Roger is an author, biohacker, podcaster and fitness entrepreneur, with an eye firmly on research and innovation.

In his pursuit of physical and mental refinement, he has aligned himself with some of the most pioneering minds in science, nutrition and wellness.

beacons.ai/rogersnipes

RESOURCES

pp.38, 121–2, 124 www.britannica.com/science/adenosine-triphosphate

pp.78–9 P. Arner, S. Bernard, L. Appelsved, K.-Y. Fu, D. P. Andersson, M. Salehpour, A. Thorell, M. Rydén, K. L. Spalding. *Adipose lipid turnover and long-term changes in body weight*. Nature Medicine, (2019)

p.84 www.ncbi.nlm.nih.gov/pmc/articles/PMC5513193/

p.87 www.healthline.com/nutrition/thermogenics#what-are-they

p.87 www.nhs.uk/live-well/healthy-weight/bmi-calculator/

p.88 www.active.com/fitness/calculators/bmr

p.95, 157 www.dietdoctor.com/fasting-and-growth-hormone

p.113 Pollack, Gerald H. *The Fourth Phase of Water: Beyond Solid, Liquid, and Vapor.* Ebner and Sons. (2013)

p.113–14 daveasprey.com/ez-water/

p.120. www.healthline.com/health/emf#TOC_TITLE_HDR_1

p.121. www.researchsquare.com/article/rs-21211/v1

p.126 www.healthline.com/nutrition/bovine-colostrum#what-it-is

p.127 www.bulletproof.com/recipes

p.128 www.health.harvard.edu/blog/apple-cider-vinegar-diet-does-it-really-work-2018042513703

p.129 www.nhs.uk/conditions/coronavirus-covid-19/people-at-higher-risk/get-vitamin-d-supplements/

p.129 www.nutriadvanced.co.uk/news/thinking-of-supplementing-with-vitamin-d-think-vitamin-k2-too/

p.134 www.healthline.com/nutrition/hydrogen-wate

p.136 www.nuffieldhealth.com/article/what-is-aerobic-vs-anaerobic-training

p.156 www.muscleandfitness.com/workouts/full-body-exercises/top-10-compound-lifts-maximum-size-and-strength/

p.157 link.springer.com/article/10.1007/s004210050323

p.157 *European Journal of Applied Physiology and Occupational Physiology*

INDEX